POCKET GUIDE TO DRUG INTERACTIONS

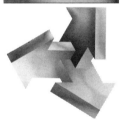

 LIPPINCOTT WILLIAMS & WILKINS

A **Wolters Kluwer** Company

Philadelphia • Baltimore • New York • London
Buenos Aires • Hong Kong • Sydney • Tokyo

Staff

Editorial Director
William J. Kelly

Clinical Director
Marguerite S. Ambrose, RN, MSN, CS

Creative Director
Jake Smith

Art Director
Elaine Kasmer

Drug Information Editor
Melissa M. Devlin, PharmD

Associate Editor
Anne Stuart Dawson

Clinical Project Editor
Eileen Cassin Gallen, RN, BSN

Clinical Editor
Kimberly A. Zalewski, RN, MSN, CEN

Copy Editors
Leslie Dworkin, Dolores Connors Matthews, Jane Smith, Jenifer F. Walker

Designers
Arlene Putterman (associate design director), Joseph John Clark, Jan Greenberg, Donald G. Knauss

Typographers
Diane Paluba (manager), Joyce Rossi Biletz

Manufacturing
Patricia K. Dorshaw (manager), Beth Janae Orr (book production manager)

Editorial Assistants
Danielle J. Barsky, Carol A. Caputo, Arlene P. Claffee

Indexer
Barbara Hodgson

Contents

Clinical consultants

Tricia M. Berry, PharmD, BCPS
Assistant Professor of Pharmacy Practice
St. Louis College of Pharmacy
St. Louis, Mo.

Lawrence Carey, PharmD
Clinical Pharmacist Supervisor
Jefferson Home Infusion Service
Philadelphia, Pa.

Robert Lee Page II, PharmD, BCPS
Assistant Professor
University of Colorado Health Sciences
    Center, School of Pharmacy
Denver, Colo.

Gary Smith, RPh, PharmD
Manager, Clinical Pharmacy Services
Fairview Physician Associates
Edina, Minn.

Joseph F. Steiner, RPh, PharmD
Professor and Director of Pharmacy
    Practice
University of Wyoming School of Pharmacy
Laramie, Wyo.

Tatyana Gurvich, PharmD
Clinical Pharmacologist
Glendale Adventist Family Residency
    Program
Glendale, Calif.

AnhThu Hoang, PharmD
Medical Director
IntraMed Educational Group
New York, N.Y.

Christine Price, PharmD
Clinical Coordinator
Department of Pharmacology Services
Morton Plant Meare Health Care
Dunedin, Fla.

Susan W. Sard, PharmD
Clinical Pharmacist
Anne Arundel Medical Center
Annapolis, MD
Clinical Instructor
Anne Arundel Community College
Annapolis, Md.

How to use this book

NDH Pocket Guide to Drug Interactions gives you a quick resource for drug interactions.

The book is organized alphabetically by primary generic drug names, which appear in a shaded bar above three columns of interaction information. Next to each primary generic name, you'll find common trade names. Canadian trade names are denoted by a dagger (†).

The first column below the shaded bar lists the interacting agents for each primary drug. Interacting agents are drugs (generic names), herbs, foods, and lifestyle behaviors (such as smoking and drinking alcohol). Both prescription and nonprescription drugs are listed, when applicable. An interacting agent may appear more than once under a primary drug if it can produce more than one significant effect. Interactions in bold type indicate severe, well-documented interactions that may be life-threatening and should be avoided.

The second column covers possible effects that may result when the interacting agent is used concomitantly with the primary drug. These effects may be an increase in certain risks, a fluctuation of drug levels, an increase in side effects, or other complications that may arise. Keep in mind that these are only possible effects and that actual effects may vary with each patient.

The third column lists nursing considerations related to monitoring, drug administration, and patient teaching. Precautions and warnings are also listed in this column.

Appendices include normal laboratory test values and therapeutic drug monitoring guidelines.

The index contains generic names, trade names, and interacting agents.

Guide to abbreviations

ABG	arterial blood gas	DTP	diphtheria, tetanus, and pertussis
ACE	angiotensin-converting enzyme	DVT	deep vein thrombosis
ADH	antidiuretic hormone	ECG	electrocardiogram
AIDS	acquired immunodeficiency syndrome	EEG	electroencephalogram
		ET	endotracheal
ALT	alanine aminotransferase	g	gram
aPTT	activated partial thrombo-plastin time	GFR	glomerular filtration rate
		GI	gastrointestinal
AST	aspartate aminotransferase	GU	genitourinary
AV	atrioventricular	H	histamine
b.i.d.	twice a day	HbA$_{1c}$	glycosylated hemoglobin
BP	blood pressure	Hct	hematocrit
BUN	blood urea nitrogen	HDL	high-density lipoprotein
CABG	coronary artery bypass graft	Hgb	hemoglobin
CAD	coronary artery disease	HIV	human immunodeficiency virus
CBC	complete blood count		
CDC	Centers for Disease Control and Prevention	HMG-CoA	3-hydroxy-3-methylglutaryl coenzyme A
CK	creatine kinase	HR	heart rate
cm	centimeter	hr	hour
CMV	cytomegalovirus	h.s.	at bedtime
CNS	central nervous system	I&O	intake and output
COPD	chronic obstructive pulmonary disease	I.M.	intramuscular
		INR	international normalized ratio
CrCl	creatinine clearance	IOP	intraocular pressure
CSF	cerebrospinal fluid	IPPB	intermittent positive-pressure breathing
CV	cardiovascular		
CVA	cerebrovascular accident	IU	international unit
CVP	central venous pressure	I.V.	intravenous
D$_5$W	dextrose 5% in water	kg	kilogram
dl	deciliter	L	liter

Guide to abbreviations

lb	pound	PT	prothrombin time
LDL	low-density lipoprotein	PTCA	percutaneous transluminal coronary angioplasty
LFT	liver function test		
M	molar	PTT	partial thromboplastin time
m²	square meter	PVD	peripheral vascular disease
MAC	*Mycobacterium avium* complex	q	every
		q.d.	every day
MAO	monoamine oxidase	q.i.d.	four times a day
MAOI	monoamine oxidase inhibitor	RBC	red blood cell
mcg	microgram	RDA	recommended daily allowance
mEq	milliequivalent		
mg	milligram	SaO₂	oxygen saturation
MI	myocardial infarction	S.C.	subcutaneous
min	minute	sec	second
ml	milliliter	S.L.	sublingual
mm³	cubic millimeter	SSRI	selective serotonin reuptake inhibitor
mo	month		
NaCl	sodium chloride	T₃	triiodothyronine
NAPA	N-Acetylprocainamide	T₄	thyroxine
NG	nasogastric	TB	tuberculosis
NSAID	nonsteroidal anti-inflammatory drug	TCA	tricyclic antidepressant
		t.i.d.	three times a day
O₂	oxygen	TPN	total parenteral nutrition
OTC	over-the-counter	tsp	teaspoon
PABA	para-aminobenzoic acid	U	unit
PAWP	pulmonary artery wedge pressure	USP	United States Pharmacopeia
		UTI	urinary tract infection
P.O.	by mouth	WBC	white blood cell
P.R.	per rectum	wk	week
p.r.n.	as needed	yr	year
PSVT	paroxysmal supraventricular tachycardia		

INTERACTING AGENTS	POSSIBLE EFFECTS	NURSING CONSIDERATIONS
abacavir sulfate • Ziagen		
alcohol	May reduce elimination of abacavir, increasing overall exposure to drug.	• Advise patient to avoid alcohol.
abciximab • ReoPro		
anticoagulants antiplatelet drugs heparin NSAIDs thrombolytics	May increase risk of bleeding.	• Monitor patient closely for increased bleeding or bruising tendencies. • Monitor CBC, PT, PTT, and INR carefully.
acarbose • Precose		
calcium channel blockers corticosteroids estrogens isoniazid nicotinic acid oral contraceptives phenothiazines phenytoin sympathomimetics thiazides, other diuretics thyroid hormones	May cause hyperglycemia or hypoglycemia when withdrawn.	• Monitor serum glucose level closely. • Monitor patient carefully for signs of hypoglycemia, including dizziness, diaphoresis, confusion, and tachycardia. • Monitor patient for signs of hyperglycemia, including fatigue, polyuria, polydipsia, weight loss, abdominal pain, altered mental status, tachycardia, hypotension, glucosuria, and ketonuria. • Dosage adjustment may be needed after concurrent therapy.
digestive enzyme preparations containing carbohydrate-splitting enzymes (amylase, pancreatin) intestinal adsorbents (activated charcoal)	May reduce the effect of acarbose.	• Don't give these drugs together. Give acarbose at least 1 hr before or 2 hr after other drugs.
insulin sulfonylureas	May increase the hypoglycemic potential of these drugs.	• Monitor blood glucose level closely. • Monitor patient carefully for signs of hypoglycemia, including dizziness, di-

aphoresis, confusion, and tachycardia.

acetaminophen • Acephen, Anacin Aspirin Free, Feverall, Panadol, Tempra, Tylenol

anticoagulants thrombolytics	May potentiate effects of these drugs, but this appears to be clinically insignificant.	• Monitor PT and INR routinely.
antacids	May delay and decrease acetaminophen's absorption.	• Separate administration times. Administer acetaminophen dose at least 1 hr before or 2 hr after the antacid.
alcohol anticonvulsants isoniazid	May increase risk of hepatotoxicity.	• Use together cautiously. • Monitor liver function test results. • Monitor patient for signs of hepatotoxicity (jaundice, fever, abdominal pain, clay-colored stools, tea-colored urine). • Discourage alcohol use.
phenothiazines	If used with acetaminophen in large doses, hypothermia may result.	• Use together cautiously. • Monitor patient for adverse effects, such as an altered level of consciousness or change in baseline vital signs.
feverfew ginkgo biloba	May pose a risk of bleeding.	• Advise patient not to use together. • Advise patient to contact a health care professional before using herbal preparations.
red clover	Effects of red clover may enhance anticoagulation.	• Advise patient not to use together. • Monitor PT and INR closely. • Advise patient to contact health care professional before using herbal preparations.

(continued)

INTERACTING AGENTS	POSSIBLE EFFECTS	NURSING CONSIDERATIONS
acetaminophen (continued)		
watercress	May inhibit oxidative metabolism of acetaminophen.	• Advise patient not to use together. • Advise patient to contact a health care professional before using herbal preparations.
food	May delay and decrease absorption of acetaminophen.	• Advise patient to take drug on an empty stomach.
acyclovir (acycloguanosine) **acyclovir sodium)** • Zovirax		
probenecid	May reduce renal tubular secretion of acyclovir, leading to increased drug half-life, reduced elimination rate, and decreased urine excretion. Reduced clearance may cause more sustained serum drug levels.	• The dosage of acyclovir may have to be reduced if toxicity develops.
methotrexate	May cause reaction in patients who have had a previous neurologic reaction to intrathececal methotrexate.	• Use I.V. acyclovir with caution.
zidovudine	May increase levels of acyclovir, causing toxicity.	• If severe lethargy or drowsiness occurs, reduce acyclovir dosage.
albuterol sulfate • Airet, Proventil, Proventil HFA, Proventil Repetabs, Proventil Syrup, Ventolin, Ventolin Syrup, Volmax		
epinephrine orally inhaled sympathomimetic amines	May increase sympathomimetic effects and risk of toxicity. Adverse CV effects include arrhythmias, severe tachycardia, chest pain, and myocardial ischemia.	• Use together cautiously for the short-term management of moderate to severe asthma p.r.n.

MAO inhibitors TCAs	Serious CV effects may occur, including tachycardia, arrhythmias, and angina-like pain.	• Use with extreme caution in patients receiving these drugs or within 2 wk of stopping these drugs.
beta blockers propranolol	May antagonize the effects of albuterol and cause severe bronchospasm in asthmatic patients.	• Don't use together; or use cardioselective beta blockers if needed.

alendronate sodium • Fosamax

antacids calcium supplements	May interfere with alendronate absorption.	• Have patient wait at least 30 min after alendronate dose before taking other drugs.
aspirin NSAIDs	May increase risk of upper GI tract reaction with alendronate doses > 10 mg/day.	• Monitor patient closely for nausea, dyspepsia, abdominal pain, or gastritis.
hormone replacement agents	Not recommended when used with alendronate in treating osteoporosis; evidence of effectiveness is lacking.	• Don't use together.
food	May decrease absorption of alendronate.	• Don't give drug with food.

allopurinol • Purinol†, Zyloprim
allopurinol sodium • Aloprim

thiazide diuretics	In patients with decreased renal function, there may be an increased risk of allopurinol-induced hypersensitivity reactions.	• Use together cautiously and monitor patient for symptoms of hypersensitivity reactions (fever, chills, pruritus, rash).
azathioprine **mercaptopurine**	May increase the toxic effects of these drugs, particularly bone marrow depression.	• Initial doses of azathioprine or mercaptopurine need to be reduced by 25% to 33%. • Subsequent doses need to be adjusted according to response and toxic effects.

(continued)

INTERACTING AGENTS	POSSIBLE EFFECTS	NURSING CONSIDERATIONS
allopurinol (continued)		
cyclophosphamide	May increase risk of bone marrow depression.	• Frequently monitor CBC.
dicumarol	Allopurinol may inhibit hepatic microsomal metabolism of dicumarol, increasing its half-life.	• Observe for increased anticoagulant effects and adjust anticoagulant p.r.n.
amoxicillin ampicillin	May increase the risk of rash.	• Be alert for allergic-type rashes. • The dose of allopurinol may need to be lowered or the drug stopped.
chlorpropamide	Allopurinol or its metabolites may compete with chlorpropamide for renal tubular secretion.	• Observe patient for signs of excessive hypoglycemia (dizziness, diaphoresis, confusion, tachycardia).
co-trimoxazole	Use with allopurinol has been associated with thrombocytopenia.	• Monitor CBC and platelet count.
theophylline	Theophylline clearance may decrease with large doses (600 mg/day), leading to an increase in serum theophylline level.	• Monitor theophylline serum level closely and adjust dosage p.r.n. to avoid toxicity. • Signs of toxicity include tachycardia, nausea, vomiting, diarrhea, restlessness, headaches, agitation, palpitations, and arrhythmias.
alprazolam • Alprazolam Intensol, Apo-Alpraz†, Novo-Alprazol†, Xanax		
alcohol antidepressants antihistamines barbiturates general anesthetics MAO inhibitors	Alprazolam may potentiate the CNS-depressant effects of these agents.	• Monitor patient closely for increased sedation or other signs of CNS depression. • Alprazolam dose may need to be decreased or dosing interval extended. • Advise patient to avoid alcohol.

narcotics
phenothiazines

cimetidine disulfiram	May diminish hepatic metabolism of alprazolam, increasing its plasma level.	• Monitor patient for increased sedation. • Alprazolam dose may need to be decreased or dosing interval extended.
haloperidol	Alprazolam may decrease serum level of haloperidol.	• Monitor patient for clinical effects of haloperidol.
digoxin	Serum level of digoxin may increase.	• Monitor serum digoxin level.
rifampin	The effects of alprazolam may decrease.	• Monitor patient for clinical effect. • Dosage adjustment may be needed.
theophylline	May decrease the sedative effects of alprazolam.	• Monitor patient for clinical effect. • Dosage adjustment may be needed.
kava	May induce coma if taken with alprazolam.	• Advise patient not to use together.
smoking (heavy)	May accelerate alprazolam metabolism, lowering clinical effectiveness.	• Discourage smoking.

aluminum carbonate • Basaljel

| **tetracyclines**
antimuscarinics
chlordiazepoxide
coumarin anticoagulants
diazepam
digoxin
indomethacin
iron salts
isoniazid
phenothiazines (especially chlorpromazine)
quinolones
sodium or potassium phosphate | Aluminum carbonate may decrease absorption of many drugs by changing the GI transit time or by binding or forming an insoluble chelate with the drugs, thereby lessening their effectiveness. | • Recommend separating administration times by at least 2 hr; in the case of tetracyclines, separate administration times by 3 to 4 hr.
• Monitor patient for expected clinical effects of drug.
• Monitor serum drug levels or clinical effects if applicable. |

(continued)

Interacting agents in **bold type** indicate severe, well-documented interactions.   †Canadian

INTERACTING AGENTS	POSSIBLE EFFECTS	NURSING CONSIDERATIONS
aluminum carbonate *(continued)*		
enterically coated drugs	May cause premature drug release.	• Separate administration by at least 2 hr.
amiodarone hydrochloride • Cordarone		
beta blockers calcium channel blockers	May cause sinus bradycardia, sinus arrest, and AV block.	• Monitor patient closely for cardiotoxicity, especially when giving initial loading doses of amiodarone.
cholestyramine	May increase elimination of amiodarone.	• Monitor patient for decreased clinical effects.
cimetidine	May increase amiodarone level.	• Monitor amiodarone serum level when initiating cimetidine. • Dosage adjustment may be needed.
cyclosporine **digoxin** flecainide lidocaine phenytoin procainamide **quinidine** theophylline	May lead to increased serum levels of these drugs, resulting in enhanced effects and toxicity.	• Monitor drug levels. • Monitor patient for signs of toxicity (prolonged QT or QRS intervals, arrhythmias, visual disturbances, seizures, nystagmus, ataxia, lethargy). • Dosage adjustment may be needed.
general anesthetics	Serious cardiac and CV effects may occur.	• Close perioperative monitoring is needed; amiodarone may sensitize patients to adverse CV effects associated with general anesthetics.
phenytoin	May decrease amiodarone level.	• Monitor patient for loss of clinical effect and adjust dose as appropriate.

disopyramide phenothiazines pimozide **quinidine** sparfloxacin TCAs	May cause additive effects that lead to a prolonged QT interval, possibly resulting in torsades de pointes ventricular tachycardia.	• Quinolones are contraindicated in combination with amiodarone. • Use other drugs with caution and closely monitor cardiac rhythm, ECG, and serum drug levels p.r.n.
warfarin	May cause prolonged PT as a result of enhanced drug displacement from protein-binding sites.	• Monitor PT and INR closely. • A 30% to 50% reduction in the warfarin dose may be needed.
pennyroyal	Amiodarone may change the rate of formation of toxic metabolites of pennyroyal.	• Discourage use together.
sunlight exposure	Photosensitivity reactions may result.	• Advise patient to use sunblock.
amitriptyline hydrochloride • Amitriptyline, Elavil, Levate†, Novotriptyn†		
antihistamines antiparkinsonians atropine meperidine phenothiazines	May cause oversedation, hyperthermia, paralytic ileus, visual changes, and severe constipation.	• Monitor clinical effects closely and adjust dosing p.r.n.
barbiturates smoking (heavy)	May induce metabolism of amitriptyline and decrease therapeutic efficacy.	• Monitor clinical effects. • Amitriptyline dosage adjustment may be needed. • Discourage smoking.
centrally acting antihypertensives (such as guanethidine, guanabenz, guanadrel, **clonidine**, methyldopa, reserpine)	May decrease hypotensive effects of these drugs.	• Don't use clonidine with amitriptyline. • Monitor BP closely during first few weeks of concomitant therapy. • May need to use alternative antihypertensive to control BP.

(continued)

Interacting agents in **bold type** indicate severe, well-documented interactions.   †Canadian

INTERACTING AGENTS	POSSIBLE EFFECTS	NURSING CONSIDERATIONS

amitriptyline hydrochloride *(continued)*

INTERACTING AGENTS	POSSIBLE EFFECTS	NURSING CONSIDERATIONS
CNS depressants (such as alcohol, analgesics, barbiturates, narcotics, tranquilizers, anesthetics)	May cause additive CNS and respiratory effects, including oversedation.	• Monitor clinical effects closely. Give 2 hr apart to decrease sedative effects. • Advise patient to avoid alcohol.
disulfiram ethchlorvynol	May cause delirium, psychoses, and acute organic brain syndrome. The bioavailability of amitriptyline may be increased by disulfiram.	• Monitor patient closely. • Reduced dosages may be needed.
beta blockers cimetidine methylphenidate oral contraceptives propoxyphene SSRIs (such as Prozac)	May inhibit amitriptyline metabolism, increasing plasma level and toxicity.	• Use together cautiously. • Monitor patient for signs of toxicity, including sedation, lethargy, lightheadedness, memory impairment, psychomotor retardation, dry mouth, and constipation.
metrizamide	May increase risk of seizures.	• Don't use together.
MAO inhibitors	Hyperpyretic crises, seizures, and death may occur.	• Don't give with or within 2 wk of MAO inhibitor therapy.
haloperidol phenothiazines	May decrease amitriptyline's metabolism, decreasing therapeutic efficacy.	• Be prepared to adjust dosages of these drugs.
sympathomimetics (such as epinephrine, phenylephrine, ephedrine)	Amitriptyline potentiates the pressor response of these drugs and may cause arrhythmias and hypertension.	• Monitor patient for arrhythmias and hypertension.
antiarrhythmics (quinidine, disopyramide, procainamide) pimozide thyroid hormones	May increase risk of arrhythmias and conduction defects.	• Monitor ECG and cardiac rhythm closely.

warfarin	May increase PT and INR and cause bleeding.	• Monitor PT and INR. • Warfarin dosage may need to be lowered.
sun exposure	Photosensitivity reactions may result.	• Advise patient to use sunblock.

amlodipine besylate • Norvasc

grapefruit juice	May elevate amlodipine level, increasing its pharmacologic and adverse effects.	• Don't give with grapefruit juice.

amoxapine • Asendin

atropine or other anticholinergics (including phenothiazines, antihistamines, meperidine, antiparkinsonians)	May cause oversedation, paralytic ileus, visual changes, and severe constipation.	• Monitor patient for increased sedation, respiratory depression, and GI and visual complaints. • Dosage adjustment may be needed. • Advise patient to avoid alcohol.
barbiturates	May induce amoxapine metabolism and decrease therapeutic efficacy.	• Monitor patient for increased sedation or respiratory depression. • Dosage adjustment may be needed.
centrally acting antihypertensives (such as guanethidine, guanabenz, guanadrel, **clonidine,** methyldopa, reserpine)	Amoxapine may decrease hypotensive effects.	• Don't use with clonidine. • When used with other drugs, monitor BP frequently, especially at start of therapy. Alternative antihypertensives may be needed.
CNS depressants (including analgesics, barbiturates, narcotics, tranquilizers, anesthetics)	May increase sedation.	• Use together cautiously. • Monitor patient for increased sedation, dizziness, agitation, asthenia, or respiratory depression.
disulfiram ethchlorvynol	May cause delirium and tachycardia.	• Observe patient closely for these adverse effects or other signs of psychosis.

(continued)

Interacting agents in **bold type** indicate severe, well-documented interactions.   †Canadian

INTERACTING AGENTS	POSSIBLE EFFECTS	NURSING CONSIDERATIONS
amoxapine (continued)		
beta blockers cimetidine methylphenidate oral contraceptives propoxyphene	May inhibit amoxapine metabolism, increasing plasma levels.	• Monitor for signs of toxicity, including excessive anticholinergic effects (agitation, irritation, confusion, hallucinations, hyperthermia, parkinsonian symptoms, seizures, urine retention, dry mucous membranes, pupillary dilation, constipation, ileus). • CNS-depressant effects may follow, including hypothermia, decreased reflexes, sedation, hypotension, cyanosis, and conduction abnormalities.
evening primrose oil metrizamide	May increase risk of seizures.	• Don't use together, if possible. • Monitor patient closely for increased seizures. • Advise patient to contact a health care professional before using herbs.
phenothiazines haloperidol	May decrease metabolism, reducing therapeutic efficacy.	• Monitor patient for clinical effects and signs of toxicity. • Dosage adjustment may be needed.
sympathomimetics (including epinephrine, phenylephrine, ephedrine [often found in nasal sprays])	May increase BP.	• Patient needs frequent BP checks. • Monitor patient for severe hypertension.
antiarrhythmics (quinidine, disopyramide, procainamide) pimozide thyroid hormones	May increase incidence of arrhythmias and conduction defects.	• Monitor ECG closely when concurrent drug therapy starts.
MAO inhibitors	Hyperpyretic crises, seizures, and death may occur.	• Don't administer amoxapine with or within 2 wk of MAO inhibitor therapy.

quinolones	May potentiate life-threatening cardiac arrhythmias.	• Don't use together.
warfarin	May prolong PT and cause bleeding.	• Monitor PT and INR. • Dosage adjustment may be needed.
smoking (heavy)	May induce amoxapine metabolism and decrease therapeutic efficacy.	• Discourage smoking.
sun exposure	Photosensitivity reactions may result.	• Advise patient to use sunblock.

amoxicillin/clavulanate potassium • Augmentin, Clavulin†

allopurinol	May increase risk of rash from both drugs.	• Don't use together, if possible.
probenecid	May block tubular secretion of amoxicillin, raising serum level; it has no effect on clavulanate.	• Probenecid may be used for this purpose.
methotrexate	Large doses of amoxicillin may interfere with renal tubular secretion of methotrexate, delaying elimination and prolonging elevated serum level of methotrexate.	• Monitor patient for methotrexate toxicity; monitor serum levels. • An alternative antibiotic may be needed.
oral contraceptives	May decrease effectiveness of oral contraceptives.	• Advise patient to use barrier contraception.
tetracyclines	May reduce amoxicillin effectiveness.	• Don't use together.

amoxicillin trihydrate • Amoxil, Polymox, Trimox

allopurinol	May increase risk of rash from both drugs.	• Don't use together, if possible.
clavulanate potassium	May enhance effect of amoxicillin against certain beta-lactamase–producing bacteria.	• Drug may be used for this therapeutic effect.

(continued)

Interacting agents in **bold type** indicate severe, well-documented interactions.   †Canadian

INTERACTING AGENTS	POSSIBLE EFFECTS	NURSING CONSIDERATIONS
amoxicillin trihydrate *(continued)*		
methotrexate	Large doses of amoxicillin may interfere with renal tubular secretion of methotrexate, delaying elimination and prolonging elevated serum level of methotrexate.	• Monitor patient for methotrexate toxicity; monitor serum levels. • An alternative antibiotic may be needed.
oral contraceptives	May decrease effectiveness of oral contraceptives.	• Advise patient to use barrier contraception.
probenecid	May block renal tubular secretion of amoxicillin, raising serum level.	• Probenecid may be used for this purpose.
tetracyclines	May reduce amoxicillin effectiveness.	• Don't use together.
ampicillin • Apo-Ampi†, Novo-Ampicillin†, Omnipen, Penbritin† **ampicillin sodium** • Ampicin†, Omnipen-N, Penbritin† **ampicillin trihydrate** • Omnipen, Principen, Totacillin		
aminoglycoside antibiotic	May cause a synergistic bactericidal effect against some strains of enterococci and group B streptococci; however, the drugs are physically and chemically incompatible and are inactivated if mixed or given together.	• Don't mix together.
allopurinol	May increase risk of rash from both drugs.	• Don't use together, if possible.
clavulanate	May increase bactericidal effects because clavulanic acid is a beta-lactamase inhibitor.	• Drug may be used for this therapeutic effect.
methotrexate	Large doses of ampicillin may interfere with renal tubular secretion of metho-	• Monitor patient for methotrexate toxicity; monitor serum level.

	trexate, delaying elimination and pro- longing elevated serum level of methotrexate.	• An alternative antibiotic may be needed.
probenecid	May inhibit renal tubular secretion of ampi- cillin, raising serum level.	• Probenecid may be used for this pur- pose.
oral contraceptives	May decrease effectiveness of oral contra- ceptives.	• Advise patient to use barrier method.
tetracyclines	May reduce ampicillin effectiveness.	• Don't use together.

amprenavir • Agenerase

antiarrhythmics (such as amiodarone, lidocaine [systemic], quinidine) anticoagulants (such as warfarin) TCAs	May increase serum levels of these drugs.	• Monitor patient for increased clinical ef- fects and signs of toxicity. • Monitor serum drug levels.
grapefruit juice macrolides	May increase amprenavir plasma level.	• Monitor patient for signs of toxicity. • Dose adjustment may be needed. • Drug should be taken with liquid other than grapefruit juice.
psychotherapeutics	May cause increased CNS effects.	• Monitor patient closely for increased se- dation, dizziness, ataxia, tremor, agita- tion, and respiratory depression.
rifabutin	May decrease amprenavir level and cause a substantial increase in rifabutin level.	• Monitor patient for clinical effectiveness. • Rifabutin dosage may need to be re- duced.
sildenafil	May substantially increase sildenafil level, which may increase sildenafil-associated effects, including hypotension, visual changes, and priapism.	• Use together very cautiously; sildenafil should be given in reduced dosages.

(continued)

INTERACTING AGENTS	POSSIBLE EFFECTS	NURSING CONSIDERATIONS
amprenavir *(continued)*		
bepridil dihydroergotamine midazolam rifampin triazolam	Competition for CYP3A4 by amprenavir may inhibit the metabolism of midazolam and triazolam and create the potential for serious or life-threatening events, such as arrhythmias or prolonged sedation. Rifampin is a potent inducer of CYP3A4, which could markedly diminish plasma levels of amprenavir. There is an increased risk of ergot toxicity (peripheral vasospasm, ischemia of the extremities). Amprenavir may substantially increase bepridil serum level with an associated increase in adverse effects.	• Don't give together
antacids high-fat meals	May decrease absorption of amprenavir.	• Separate administration of antacids and drug by at least 1 hr. • Advise patient not to take drug with a high-fat meal.
St. John's wort	May decrease amprenavir level. May decrease blood level of indinavir by an average of 57%. This may lead to failure of the drug to keep HIV in check. Similar effects are expected to occur with other protease inhibitors.	• Discourage use together. • Advise patient to contact a health care professional before using herbal preparations.
ascorbic acid (vitamin C) • Cecon, Cevi-Bid, Ce-Vi-Sol, Dull-C, Vita-C		
acidic drugs in large doses (more than 2 g/day)	May lower urine pH, causing renal tubular reabsorption of acidic drugs.	• Monitor patient for clinical and adverse effects.

iron	Ascorbic acid maintains iron in the ferrous state and increases iron absorption in the GI tract, but this increase may not be significant.	• A combination of 30 mg of iron and 200 mg of ascorbic acid is recommended.
dicumarol	May influence intensity and duration of the anticoagulant effect.	• Monitor patient for increased bleeding tendencies. Monitor PT and INR.
warfarin	May inhibit the anticoagulant effect.	• Monitor PT and INR.
ethinyl estradiol	May increase serum level of ethinyl estradiol.	• Monitor serum level of this drug.
salicylates	May inhibit ascorbic acid uptake by leukocytes and platelets.	• Observe patient for symptoms of ascorbic acid deficiency, including muscle weakness, anemia, edema, softening of the gums with ulcerations and loosened teeth, poor wound healing, and mucocutaneous hemorrhage.
smoking	May decrease serum ascorbic acid level, increasing dosage requirements of this vitamin.	• Advise patient to avoid heavy smoking, especially if he has a deficiency of vitamin C.

aspirin • A.S.A., Ascriptin, Aspergum, Bufferin, Ecotrin, Empirin, Halfprin, Novasen†, ZORprin

anticoagulants thrombolytics	May potentiate the platelet-inhibiting effects of aspirin.	• Monitor patient for increased bleeding tendencies. Monitor PT, PTT, and INR.
phenytoin sulfonylureas **warfarin**	May cause displacement of either drug and lead to adverse effects.	• Monitor for clinical effect and toxicity. • Monitor serum phenytoin level, serum glucose, PT, and INR as appropriate. • Consider recommending an alternative drug.

(continued)

INTERACTING AGENTS	POSSIBLE EFFECTS	NURSING CONSIDERATIONS
aspirin (continued)		
ketorolac	May increase risk of serious ketorolac adverse effects.	• Avoid using together.
methotrexate	May increase toxic effects of methotrexate.	• Monitor patient for signs of toxicity, including myelosuppression, anemia, nausea, vomiting, diarrhea, dermatitis, alopecia, melena, and fatigue. • Monitor serum levels.
alcohol antibiotics NSAIDs	May potentiate the adverse GI effects of aspirin.	• Monitor patient for GI complaints. • Advise patient to avoid alcohol.
aminoglycosides bumetanide capreomycin cisplatin erythromycin ethacrynic acid furosemide vancomycin	May potentiate ototoxic effects.	• Advise patient of this potential interaction. • Avoid this combination, if possible. • If used together, perform a baseline hearing test and monitor periodically thereafter. • Dosage adjustment or withdrawal of a drug may be needed.
lithium	Aspirin may decrease renal clearance of lithium carbonate, increasing serum lithium level and the risk of adverse effects.	• Monitor serum lithium level. • Look for signs of toxicity, including sedation, confusion, tremors, muscle stiffness, increased deep tendon reflexes, visual changes, and nystagmus.
phenylbutazone probenecid sulfinpyrazone	Aspirin may antagonize the uricosuric effect of these drugs.	• Advise patient to avoid products that contain aspirin when taking these drugs.

ammonium chloride urine acidifiers	May increase aspirin blood levels.	• Monitor patient for signs of aspirin toxicity, including lethargy, tinnitus, GI discomfort, oliguria, acute renal failure, hyperthermia, tachypnea, acid-base imbalance, dehydration, pulmonary edema, and tachycardia.
antacids in high doses other urine alkalizers	May decrease aspirin blood levels.	• Monitor patient for clinical effects. • Dosage adjustments may be needed at the start or end of drug therapy.
corticosteroids	May enhance aspirin elimination. May potentiate adverse GI effects of aspirin.	• Monitor patient for decreased salicylate effect and GI complaints.
feverfew ginkgo horse chestnut kelpware prickly ash red clover	May increase risk of bleeding.	• Advise patient not to use together. • Advise patient to contact a health care professional before using herbal preparations.
red clover	Coumarin effects may enhance anticoagulation.	• Advise patient not to use together. • Monitor PT and INR closely. • Advise patient to contact a health care professional before using herbal preparations.
food	May delay and decrease absorption of aspirin.	• Monitor for decreased salicylate effect.
atenolol • Tenormin		
antihypertensives	Atenolol may potentiate the antihypertensive effects of other antihypertensives.	• Monitor BP.

(continued)

INTERACTING AGENTS	POSSIBLE EFFECTS	NURSING CONSIDERATIONS
atenolol *(continued)*		
insulin oral hypoglycemics	May increase hypoglycemic effects of these drugs.	• Monitor serum glucose level. • Drug may mask the signs of excessive hypoglycemia (dizziness, diaphoresis, confusion, tachycardia).
alpha blockers (such those in OTC cold remedies) indomethacin NSAIDs	May antagonize antihypertensive effects of atenolol.	• Don't use together, if possible. • Monitor BP. • Dosage adjustment may be needed.
verapamil	May cause additive effects of both drugs.	• Monitor cardiac function. • Dosage adjustment may be needed.
atorvastatin calcium • Lipitor		
azole antifungals cyclosporine erythromycin fibric acid derivatives niacin	May increase atorvastatin serum level and increase adverse effects. May increase risk of rhabdomyolysis (skeletal muscle destruction, muscle aches, weakness).	• Don't use together, if possible. • If concurrent use is necessary, monitor patient. • Atorvastatin dose may be reduced.
antacids	May decrease level of atorvastatin. LDL-cholesterol reduction not affected.	• Monitor patient. • Separate administration times by 2 hr.
digoxin	May increase serum digoxin level.	• Monitor serum digoxin level.
grapefruit juice	May increase atorvastatin serum level and increase adverse effects, such as rhabdomyolysis (skeletal muscle destruction, muscle aches, weakness).	• Don't give together.
oral contraceptives	May increase hormone levels.	• Advise patient to consider effects when selecting an oral contraceptive.

azithromycin • Zithromax

aluminum- and magnesium-containing antacids	May cause lower peak plasma level of azithromycin.	• Separate administration times by at least 2 hr.
theophylline	Azithromycin may increase plasma theophylline level by decreasing theophylline clearance.	• Monitor theophylline levels carefully.
drugs metabolized by the hepatic cytochrome P-450 system (such as phenytoin, barbiturates, carbamazepine, cyclosporine)	May impair metabolism of these drugs and increase risk of toxicity.	• Monitor patient for signs of drug toxicity, such as increased sedation, respiratory depression, ataxia, nystagmus, arrhythmias, nausea, vomiting, tremor, and seizures. Monitor serum drug levels if available.
triazolam	May decrease clearance of triazolam, increasing the risk of triazolam toxicity.	• Monitor patient for signs of drug toxicity (increased sedation, respiratory depression, hypotension, bradycardia, hypoactive reflexes).

baclofen • Lioresal

antidiabetics insulin	Baclofen may increase serum glucose level.	• Monitor serum glucose level. • Check for signs of hyperglycemia (fatigue, polyuria, polydipsia, weight loss, abdominal pain, altered mental status, tachycardia, hypotension, glucosuria, ketonuria). • Dosage adjustment may be needed.
alcohol CNS-depressant drugs (including narcotics, antipsychotics, anxiolytics, general anesthetics)	May add to the CNS effects of drug.	• Check for signs of increased CNS depression, including increased sedation, headache, dizziness, ataxia, confusion, agitation, and respiratory depression. • Advise patient to avoid alcohol.

(continued)

INTERACTING AGENTS	POSSIBLE EFFECTS	NURSING CONSIDERATIONS
baclofen *(continued)*		
MAO inhibitors TCAs	May cause CNS depression, respiratory depression, and hypotension.	• Don't use together.
benazepril hydrochloride • Lotensin		
allopurinol	May increase risk of hypersensitivity reaction.	• Use together cautiously and monitor patient for symptoms of hypersensitivity reaction (fever, chills, pruritus, rash).
digoxin	May increase serum digoxin level.	• Monitor digoxin level. Monitor patient for signs of digoxin toxicity, including fatigue, asthenia, dizziness, arrhythmias, visual disturbances, nausea, vomiting, and diarrhea.
antihypertensives diuretics	May increase risk of excessive hypotension.	• Monitor BP. Diuretic may need to be stopped or benazepril dose lowered.
lithium	May increase serum lithium level and lithium toxicity.	• Monitor serum lithium level and monitor patient for signs of toxicity, including sedation, confusion, tremors, muscle stiffness, increased deep tendon reflexes, visual changes, and nystagmus.
potassium-sparing diuretics potassium supplements potassium-containing sodium substitutes	May pose a risk of hyperkalemia.	• Monitor renal function and serum potassium level. • Monitor patient for signs of hyperkalemia, including ECG changes, muscle weakness or flaccidity, and respiratory distress.
capsaicin	May increase risk of cough.	• Discourage using together. • Advise patient to consult a health care provider before using herbal preparations.

benztropine mesylate • Cogentin

amantadine	May amplify adverse anticholinergic effects, such as confusion and hallucinations.	• Decrease benztropine dosage before giving amantadine.
haloperidol phenothiazines	May decrease their effect, possibly reflecting direct CNS antagonism.	• Monitor patient for clinical effect.
phenothiazines	May increase the risk of adverse anticholinergic effects.	• Monitor patient for adverse effects. • Reduced phenothiazine dose may be needed.
alcohol CNS depressants	May increase the sedative effects of benztropine.	• Use together cautiously. • Monitor patient closely for increased CNS depressant effects (sedation, dizziness, ataxia, tremor, agitation, respiratory depression). • Advise patient to avoid alcohol.
antacids antidiarrheals	May decrease benztropine absorption.	• Give benztropine at least 1 hr before giving these drugs.

bepridil hydrochloride • Vascor

beta blockers	May cause excessive bradycardia and conduction abnormalities.	• Use together cautiously. • Monitor vital signs and ECG rhythm.
digoxin	May cause modest increases in steady-state serum digoxin level.	• Monitor serum digoxin level.
potassium-wasting diuretics	May cause hypokalemia, which increases risk of serious ventricular arrhythmias.	• Monitor serum potassium level. • Monitor patient for signs of hypokalemia, including muscle weakness, fatigue, nausea, vomiting, constipation, respiratory depression, and arrhythmias.

(continued)

INTERACTING AGENTS	POSSIBLE EFFECTS	NURSING CONSIDERATIONS
bepridil hydrochloride *(continued)*		
procainamide quinidine TCAs	May cause additive prolongation of QT interval.	• Avoid using together, if possible. • Monitor ECG for arrhythmias. Monitor QT interval closely.
biperiden hydrochloride **biperiden lactate** • Akineton		
amantadine	May amplify adverse anticholinergic effects, such as confusion and hallucinations.	• Decrease biperiden dosage before giving amantadine.
haloperidol phenothiazines	May decrease their effect, possibly reflecting direct CNS antagonism.	• Monitor patient for clinical effect.
phenothiazines	May increase the risk of adverse anticholinergic effects.	• Monitor patient for adverse effects. • Reduced phenothiazine dose may be needed.
alcohol CNS depressants	May increase the sedative effects of biperiden.	• Use together cautiously. • Monitor patient closely for increased CNS depressant effects (sedation, dizziness, ataxia, tremor, agitation, respiratory depression). • Advise patient to avoid alcohol.
antacids antidiarrheals	May decrease biperiden absorption.	• Give biperiden at least 1 hr before giving these drugs.
digoxin	May elevate serum digoxin level.	• Monitor digoxin level. • Monitor patient for signs of digoxin toxicity, including fatigue, asthenia, dizziness, arrhythmias, visual disturbances, nausea, vomiting, and diarrhea.

bisacodyl • Bisco-Lax, Correctol, Dulcolax, Fleet Laxative

antacids drugs that increase gastric pH levels milk	May cause premature dissolution of the enteric coating, resulting in intestinal or gastric irritation or cramping.	• Don't administer together, if possible. • Separate administration times. • Don't give drug with dairy products.

bisoprolol fumarate • Zebeta

beta blockers	May enhance beta blocker effects.	• Bisoprolol shouldn't be used with other beta blockers.
catecholamine-depleting drugs (such as reserpine or guanethidine)	May cause excessively reduced sympathetic activity.	• Monitor BP and HR.
clonidine	Bisoprolol may enhance the rebound hypertensive effect after withdrawal of clonidine.	• Stop bisoprolol for several days before clonidine withdrawal. • Monitor patient closely.
NSAIDs	May antagonize hypotensive effects.	• Monitor BP.

bumetanide • Bumex

antihypertensives diuretics	Bumetanide may potentiate hypotensive effects.	• These drugs are used to therapeutic advantage. • Dosage adjustments may be needed.
potassium-sparing diuretics (spironolactone, triamterene, amiloride)	May decrease bumetanide-induced potassium loss.	• Monitor serum potassium level.
lithium	May reduce renal clearance of lithium and increase lithium level.	• Monitor serum lithium level. • Lithium dosage may require adjustment. • Monitor patient for signs of toxicity.

(continued)

INTERACTING AGENTS	POSSIBLE EFFECTS	NURSING CONSIDERATIONS
bumetanide *(continued)*		
potassium-depleting drugs (such as steroids, amphotericin B)	May cause severe potassium loss.	• Monitor serum potassium level. • Monitor patient for signs of hypokalemia, including muscle weakness, fatigue, nausea, vomiting, constipation, respiratory depression, and arrhythmias.
dandelion indomethacin probenecid	May reduce the diuretic effect of bumetanide	• Combined use isn't recommended. • If drugs are used together, an increased dose of bumetanide may be required. • Advise patient against using with herbs.
ototoxic or nephrotoxic drugs	May result in enhanced toxicity	• Use together cautiously. • Monitor renal function test results. • Perform a baseline hearing test and monitor periodically. • May need to reduce dose or stop drug.
digoxin	Electrolyte disturbances may result in digoxin-induced arrhythmias.	• Monitor serum potassium, magnesium, and digoxin levels. • Supplements may be needed.
bupropion hydrochloride • Wellbutrin, Wellbutrin SR, Zyban		
drugs that lower the seizure threshold (antipsychotics, other antidepressants, theophylline, systemic steroids)	May increase risk of seizures.	• Use together cautiously. • Initial dosing should be low with small, gradual dose increases thereafter.
drugs metabolized by CYP2D6 (SSRIs, TCAs, beta blockers, antiarrhythmics, antipsychotics)	Bupropion may inhibit CYP2D6 isoenzyme.	• Dosage of these drugs may need to be reduced.

levodopa	May increase adverse effects.	• Initial dosing should be low with small, gradual dose increases thereafter.
MAO inhibitors	May cause bupropion toxicity.	• Don't give buproprion during or within 14 days MAO inhibitor therapy.
ritonavir	May increase serum bupropion level and risk for toxicity.	• Don't use together.
TCAs	May elevate plasma levels of TCAs.	• Monitor patient's clinical response.

buspirone hydrochloride • BuSpar

azole antifungal drugs diltiazem grapefruit juice macrolide antibiotics	May elevate serum buspirone level because these agents inhibit the CYP3A4 isoenzyme.	• Monitor the clinical response to buspirone and potential adverse effects. Adjust dose p.r.n. • Don't give with grapefruit juice.
MAO inhibitors	May elevate BP.	• Don't give buspirone during or within 14 days of MAO inhibitor therapy.
digoxin	Buspirone may displace digoxin from serum-binding sites.	• Monitor serum digoxin level.
alcohol CNS depressants	May increase CNS effects (sedation, fatigue, dizziness).	• Monitor patient for increased sedation if used with other CNS depressants. • Advise patient to avoid alcohol.
haloperidol	May increase serum haloperidol level.	• Decreased doses of haloperidol may be needed.

INTERACTING AGENTS	POSSIBLE EFFECTS	NURSING CONSIDERATIONS
calcium salts • calcium acetate • Calphron, PhosLo **calcium carbonate** • Calciday-667, Cal-Plus, Caltrate 600, Chooz, Os-Cal 500, Rolaids, Titralac, Tums, Tums E-X **calcium chloride • calcium citrate** • Citracal **calcium glubionate** • Neo-Calglucon **calcium gluceptate • calcium gluconate • calcium lactate • calcium phosphate, tribasic** • Posture		
atenolol fluoroquinolones tetracyclines	May decrease bioavailability of these drugs and calcium when oral preparations are taken together.	• Separate administration times by 3 to 4 hr.
cardiac glycosides	May increase digitalis toxicity.	• Administer calcium cautiously, if at all, to digitalized patients. • Monitor patient for signs of digoxin toxicity, including fatigue, asthenia, dizziness, arrhythmias, visual disturbances, nausea, vomiting, and diarrhea.
calcium channel blockers (verapamil)	May decrease calcium effectiveness; calcium channel blocker toxicity may be reversed by calcium salts.	• Monitor patient. • May be used therapeutically for toxicity.
phenytoin	May decrease absorption of both drugs.	• Avoid use together, if possible. • Monitor levels closely if concomitant use is required.
sodium polystyrene sulfonate	May increase risk of metabolic acidosis in patients with renal disease.	• Use together only if needed.
thiazide diuretics	May increase risk of hypercalcemia.	• Monitor serum calcium level.
foods containing oxalic acid (rhubarb, spinach), phytic acid (bran, whole cereals), and phosphorus (milk, dairy products)	May interfere with calcium absorption.	• Advise patient against taking calcium preparation with these agents.
alcohol	May affect calcium absorption.	• Advise patient to avoid caffeine-

caffeine tobacco		containing beverages, tobacco use, and alcohol.

candesartan cilexetil • Atacand

potassium-sparing diuretics potassium supplements potassium-containing salt substitutes	May result in hyperkalemia.	• Monitor renal function and serum potassium level. • Monitor patient for signs of hyperkalemia. • Advise patient to avoid potassium salt substitutes.

capecitabine • Xeloda

leucovorin	May increase level of 5-FU with enhanced toxicity.	• Monitor patient closely for signs of toxicity, including bone marrow depression, bleeding, nausea, vomiting, diarrhea, and dehydration.
antacids	May increase rate of absorption of capecitabine.	• Separate administration times. • Dosage adjustment may be needed.
coumadin	May cause altered PT and bleeding.	• Monitor PT and INR. Monitor patient for bleeding.

captopril • Capoten

antacids	May decrease the effects of captopril.	• Give drugs at least 2 hr apart.
digoxin	May increase serum digoxin level by 15% to 30%.	• Monitor serum digoxin levels. • Monitor patient for toxicity.
diuretics or other antihypertensives	May increase risk of excessive hypotension.	• The diuretic may need to be stopped or captopril dose lowered.
insulin oral antidiabetics	May increase risk of hypoglycemia when captopril therapy starts.	• Monitor serum glucose level. • Monitor patient for signs of excessive hypoglycemia (dizziness, diaphoresis, confusion, tachycardia). *(continued)*

Interacting agents in **bold type** indicate severe, well-documented interactions.   †Canadian

INTERACTING AGENTS	POSSIBLE EFFECTS	NURSING CONSIDERATIONS
captopril *(continued)*		
lithium	May increase serum lithium level and lithium toxicity.	• Monitor serum lithium level. • Check for signs of toxicity, including sedation, confusion, tremors, muscle stiffness, increased deep tendon reflexes, visual changes, and nystagmus.
potassium-sparing diuretics potassium supplements	May increase risk of hyperkalemia.	• Monitor renal function and serum potassium level. • Look for signs of hyperkalemia, including ECG changes, muscle weakness or flaccidity, and respiratory distress.
NSAIDs	May decrease the antihypertensive effect of captopril.	• Don't use together, if possible. • Monitor BP. NSAID may be stopped or another antihypertensive ordered.
black catechu	May cause additional hypotensive effects.	• Don't use together.
carbamazepine • Atretol, Carbatrol, Epitol, Tegretol		
cimetidine danazol diltiazem fluoxetine fluvoxamine grapefruit juice isoniazid **macrolides (such as erythromycin)** propoxyphene valproic acid verapamil	May increase carbamazepine blood level. May inhibit hepatic metabolism of carbamazepine.	• Danazol, propoxyphene, or macrolide antibiotics should not be given together. • Monitor carbamazepine serum level. • Monitor patient for toxicity (dizziness, ataxia, respiratory depression, arrhythmias, blood pressure changes, impaired consciousness, restlessness, abnormal reflexes, seizures, nausea, vomiting, urinary retention). • Don't give carbamazepine with grapefruit juice.
doxycycline	May decrease blood level of these drugs.	• Monitor serum drug levels or effects if

felbamate haloperidol oral contraceptives phenytoin theophylline warfarin		• applicable. • Monitor patient for decreased clinical effect. • Dosage adjustment may be needed. • Advise female patients to use barrier contraception.
lithium	May increase CNS toxicity of lithium.	• Monitor patient for signs of neurotoxicity (sedation, confusion, tremors, muscle stiffness, increased deep tendon reflexes, nystagmus, seizures).
MAO inhibitors	May increase depressant and anticholinergic effects.	• Don't use during or within 14 days of MAO inhibitor therapy.
phenobarbital phenytoin primidone	May decrease carbamazepine level.	• Monitor carbamazepine serum level. • Check for decreased clinical effect. • Dosage adjustment of carbamazepine may be needed.
psyllium seed	May inhibit GI absorption.	• Don't use together.

carisoprodol • Soma

alcohol CNS depressants	May increase CNS depression.	• Monitor patient for increased sedation, dizziness, ataxia, tremor, agitation. • Advise patient to avoid alcohol.

carteolol hydrochloride • Cartrol, Ocupress

calcium channel blockers	May increase risk of hypotension, left ventricular failure, and AV conduction disturbances.	• Use I.V. calcium antagonists cautiously. • Monitor cardiac function. • Dosage adjustment may be needed.
cardiac glycosides	May produce additive effects on slowing AV node conduction.	• Monitor patient's HR and rhythm.

(continued)

Interacting agents in **bold type** indicate severe, well-documented interactions.   †Canadian

INTERACTING AGENTS	POSSIBLE EFFECTS	NURSING CONSIDERATIONS
carteolol hydrochloride *(continued)*		
catecholamine-depleting drugs (such as reserpine, oral adrenergic blockers)	May have an additive effect and contribute to the development of hypotension or bradycardia.	• Monitor patient closely. • Monitor BP and HR.
clonidine	May cause potentially life-threatening hypertension.	• Closely monitor patient's BP during concomitant use and after one drug is discontinued.
epinephrine	May cause hypertension followed by bradycardia.	• Avoid using together, if possible. • If concurrent use is needed, monitor vital signs closely. • If use of epinephrine is anticipated, stop carteolol 3 days before using.
general anesthetics	May increase hypotensive effects.	• Carefully observe for hypotension, bradycardia, and orthostatic hypotension.
insulin oral antidiabetics	May alter hypoglycemic response.	• Monitor serum glucose level. • Drug may mask the signs of excessive hypoglycemia (dizziness, diaphoresis, confusion, tachycardia). • Dose may need adjustment.
NSAIDs	May antagonize hypotensive effects.	• Monitor BP.
sun exposure	Ophthalmic form of drug may cause photophobia.	• Advise patient to wear sunblock.
carvedilol • Coreg		
calcium channel blockers	May cause isolated conduction disturbances.	• Monitor ECG and BP.

catecholamine-depleting drugs (such as reserpine, MAO inhibitors)	May cause severe bradycardia or hypotension.	• Monitor HR and BP closely.
cimetidine	May increase bioavailability of carvedilol.	• Monitor vital signs closely.
clonidine	May potentiate BP and HR-lowering effects.	• Monitor vital signs closely. • If stopping concomitant therapy, stop carvedilol first, then gradually taper clonidine dose a few days later.
digoxin	May increase digoxin level by about 15%.	• Monitor serum digoxin level.
insulin oral antidiabetics	May enhance hypoglycemic properties.	• Monitor serum glucose levels. • Monitor patient for signs of excessive hypoglycemia (dizziness, diaphoresis, confusion, tachycardia).
rifampin	May reduce plasma level of carvedilol by 70%.	• Monitor patient for clinical effect. • Monitor vital signs.
food	May delay rate of absorption of carvedilol, but doesn't alter extent of bioavailability.	• Advise patient to take drug with food to minimize orthostatic effects.

cefaclor • Ceclor, Ceclor CD

antacids	Absorption of extended-release cefaclor may decrease if taken within 1 hr.	• Give 1 hr apart.
chloramphenicol	May cause antagonistic effect.	• Don't use together.
probenecid	May competitively inhibit renal tubular secretion of cefaclor, resulting in its higher, prolonged serum level.	• Combination may be used for this effect. Monitor patient for adverse effects.
loop diuretics nephrotoxic drugs (vancomycin, colistin, polymyxin B, aminoglycosides)	May increase the risk of nephrotoxicity.	• Don't use together, if possible. • If used together, monitor renal function.

Interacting agents in **bold type** indicate severe, well-documented interactions. †Canadian

INTERACTING AGENTS	POSSIBLE EFFECTS	NURSING CONSIDERATIONS
cefadroxil • Duricef		
probenecid	May competitively inhibit renal tubular secretion of cefadroxil, resulting in its higher, prolonged serum level.	• Combination may be used for this effect. • Monitor patient for adverse effects.
loop diuretics nephrotoxic drugs (vancomycin, colistin, polymyxin B, aminoglycosides)	May increase the risk of nephrotoxicity.	• Don't use together, if possible. • If used together, monitor renal function.
bacteriostatic drugs (chloramphenicol, erythromycin, tetracyclines)	May interfere with bactericidal activity.	• Don't use together, if possible. • If used together, monitor patient for lack of therapeutic effect.
cefdinir • Omnicef		
antacids (magnesium- and aluminum-containing) foods fortified with iron (such as infant formula) iron supplements	May decrease the rate of absorption and bioavailability of cefdinir.	• These preparations should be given 2 hr before or after cefdinir dose. • Cefdinir shouldn't be given with infant formula or other iron-rich foods.
probenecid	May inhibit the renal secretion of cefdinir.	• Combination may be used for this effect. • Monitor patient for adverse effects.
cefixime • Suprax		
carbamazepine	May elevate carbamazepine level.	• Monitor carbamazepine serum level. • Monitor patient for toxicity (dizziness, ataxia, respiratory depression, arrhythmias, blood pressure changes, impaired consciousness, restlessness, abnormal reflexes, seizures, nausea, vomiting, urinary retention).

| probenecid | May inhibit excretion and increase blood level of cefixime. | • Combination may be used for this effect.
• Monitor patient for adverse effects. |
| salicylates | May increase serum level of cefixime. | • Monitor patient for increased adverse reactions. This effect may be beneficial in certain infections. |

cefprozil • Cefzil

| aminoglycosides | May cause synergistic activity against some organisms. May increase the risk of nephrotoxicity of cefprozil. | • Don't use together, if possible.
• If used together, monitor aminoglycoside levels and renal function test results. |
| probenecid | May decrease excretion and increase blood level of cefprozil. | • Combination may be used for this effect.
• Monitor patient for adverse effects. |

cefuroxime axetil • Ceftin
cefuroxime sodium • Kefurox, Zinacef

aminoglycosides	May cause synergistic activity against some organisms and increase nephrotoxicity.	• Monitor aminoglycoside levels and renal function test results.
diuretics	May increase risk of adverse renal effects.	• Monitor renal function test results.
probenecid	May competitively inhibit renal tubular secretion of cefuroxime, resulting in its higher, prolonged serum level.	• May be used for this effect.
food	May increase absorption.	• Advise patient to take drug with food.

celecoxib • Celebrex

| alcohol
aspirin | May increase risk of ulcers.
Alcohol may increase risk of GI irritation or bleeding if celecoxib is used long-term. | • Low doses of aspirin can be used safely for prevention of CV events.
• Observe patient for signs of GI bleeding.
• Advise patient to avoid alcohol. |

(continued)

INTERACTING AGENTS	POSSIBLE EFFECTS	NURSING CONSIDERATIONS
celecoxib (continued)		
angiotensin-converting enzyme inhibitors	May diminish antihypertensive effects.	• Monitor BP.
fluconazole	May increase celecoxib level.	• May need to adjust celecoxib to minimal effective dosage.
furosemide	NSAIDs may reduce sodium excretion associated with diuretics, causing sodium retention.	• Observe patient for swelling and increased BP.
lithium	May increase lithium level.	• Monitor serum lithium level.
warfarin	May increase risk of bleeding complications.	• Monitor PT and INR. • Monitor patient for signs of bleeding.
cephalexin hydrochloride • Keftab **cephalexin monohydrate** • Biocef, Keflex, Novo-Lexin†		
probenecid	May competitively inhibit renal tubular secretion of cephalexin, resulting in its higher, prolonged serum level.	• Combination may be used for this effect. • Monitor patient for adverse effects.
loop diuretics nephrotoxic drugs (aminoglycosides, colistin, polymyxin B, vancomycin)	May increase the risk of nephrotoxicity.	• Monitor renal function. • Monitor drug levels if appropriate. • Reducing dosage or discontinuing one or both agents may be needed.
cetirizine hydrochloride • Zyrtec		
alcohol CNS depressants	May cause additive CNS effects.	• Monitor patient for increased sedation and dizziness. • Discourage alcohol use.
theophylline	May decrease clearance of cetirizine.	• Monitor patient for increased sedation.

cevimeline • Evoxac

beta blockers	May cause conduction disturbances	• Use together cautiously. • Monitor ECG.
parasympathomimetics	May cause additive effects.	• Use together cautiously. • Monitor patient for increased adverse effects, including headache, mental confusion, visual disturbances, lacrimation, sweating, respiratory distress, GI distress, arrhythmias, and shock.
drugs that inhibit CYP2D6, CYP3A4, CYP3A3	May inhibit metabolism of cevimeline.	• Monitor patient closely for increased adverse effects.

chloral hydrate • Aquachloral Supprettes, Noctec, Novo-Chlorhydrate†

antihistamines CNS depressants narcotics sedative-hypnotics tranquilizers TCAs	May add to or potentiate effects of these drugs.	• Monitor patient for increased adverse effects, including increased sedation, dizziness, agitation, asthenia, and respiratory depression.
I.V. furosemide	May cause a hypermetabolic state by displacing thyroid hormone from binding sites.	• Monitor for adverse effects if patient has received chloral hydrate in the previous 24 hr.
oral anticoagulants	May increase hypoprothrombinemic effects.	• Monitor PT and INR. • Monitor patient for signs of bleeding.
phenytoin	May increase elimination of phenytoin.	• Monitor serum phenytoin level.
alcohol	May cause vasodilation, tachycardia, sweating, and flushing in some patients.	• Advise patient to avoid alcohol.

INTERACTING AGENTS	POSSIBLE EFFECTS	NURSING CONSIDERATIONS
cholestyramine • Questran, Questran Light		
acetaminophen cardiac glycosides corticosteroids thiazide diuretics thyroid hormones	May reduce absorption of these drugs.	• Administer other drugs 1 hr before or 4 to 6 hr after cholestyramine. • Dosage adjustment is needed when cholestyramine is withdrawn to prevent high-dose toxicity.
warfarin	May decrease anticoagulant effects.	• Give drugs at least 3 hr apart. • Carefully monitor PT and INR.
cidofovir • Vistide		
nephrotoxic drugs (such as amphotericin B, aminoglycosides, foscarnet, I.V. pentamidine)	May increase nephrotoxicity.	• Avoid using together, if possible. • If used together, monitor serum drug levels and renal function tests.
St. John's wort	Has been found to decrease blood level of indinavir by an average of 57%. Similar effects may occur with other protease inhibitors, severely reducing drug's efficacy.	• Discourage patient from using herb with protease inhibitors. • Advise patient to contact a health care professional before using herbs.
cilostazol • Pletal		
diltiazem erythromycin and other macrolides grapefruit juice omeprazole strong inhibitors of CYP3A4 (such as ketoconazole, itraconazole, fluconazole, miconazole, fluvoxamine, fluoxetine, nefazodone, sertraline)	May increase peak serum level of cilostazol or one of its metabolites.	• Avoid using together, if possible. • Monitor patient for increased adverse effects, such as severe headache, diarrhea, hypotension, and cardiac arrhythmias if used together. • Don't give with grapefruit juice.
smoking	May decrease drug exposure by about 20%.	• Discourage smoking.

benzodiazepines **beta blockers (such as propranolol)** carmustine disulfiram isoniazid **lidocaine** metronidazole oral contraceptives phenytoin procainamide quinidine **theophylline** triamterene TCAs **warfarin** xanthines	Cimetidine may decrease hepatic metabolism of these drugs, increasing potential toxicity and possibly requiring dosage reduction.	• Avoid concomitant use of carmustine, procainamide, quinidine, or warfarin with cimetidine. Patients taking other drugs with cimetidine must be monitored for signs of toxicity. • A 20% to 40% reduction in theophylline dosing may be needed. • Monitor serum drug levels when appropriate (lidocaine, phenytoin, procainamide, quinidine, theophylline). In some cases, it may be appropriate to use an alternative H_2-antagonist, such as ranitidine. • Recommend barrier contraception for women taking oral contraceptives.
digoxin	Serum digoxin level may be reduced.	• Monitor serum digoxin level.
ferrous salts indomethacin ketoconazole tetracyclines	Cimetidine may decrease gastric pH, which may cause a decrease in the absorption of these agents.	• Give 1 to 2 hr apart. • In the case of ketoconazole, one drug should be stopped.
flecainide	May increase serum level of flecainide.	• Monitor ECG and BP. • Dosage adjustments may be needed.
pennyroyal	May change the rate of formation of toxic metabolites of pennyroyal.	• Discourage herb use.
yerba maté	May decrease clearance of yerba maté methylxanthines and cause toxicity.	• Use together cautiously.

(continued)

Interacting agents in **bold type** indicate severe, well-documented interactions.   †Canadian

INTERACTING AGENTS	POSSIBLE EFFECTS	NURSING CONSIDERATIONS
cimetidine *(continued)*		
smoking	May increase gastric acid secretion and worsen disease.	▪ Discourage smoking.
ciprofloxacin (systemic) • Cipro		
aluminum-, calcium-, and magnesium-containing antacid supplements iron minerals vitamins	May significantly reduce ciprofloxacin absorption.	▪ Antacids may be given safely 2 hr before or 6 hr after ciprofloxacin. ▪ Dietary supplements also should not be given with ciprofloxacin.
aminoglycosides beta-lactams	Synergistic effects may occur.	▪ Synergistic effects are unpredictable; monitor patient.
probenecid	May interfere with renal tubular secretion and result in a higher plasma level of ciprofloxacin.	▪ Combination may be used when high tissue and plasma levels are needed.
sucralfate	May reduce ciprofloxacin absorption by 50%.	▪ Give 2 hr apart.
theophylline	May increase risk of theophylline toxicity and prolong elimination half-life.	▪ Monitor serum theophylline level. ▪ Dosage adjustment may be needed.
warfarin	May enhance effects of anticoagulants.	▪ Monitor PT and INR closely. ▪ Warfarin dose adjustment may be needed.
yerba maté methylxanthines	May decrease clearance of yerba maté methylxanthines and cause toxicity.	▪ Discourage concomitant use.
sun exposure	Photosensitivity reaction may occur from sun exposure.	▪ Advise patient to use sunblock.
caffeine	Ciprofloxacin may prolong elimination half-life of caffeine.	▪ Advise patient of this interaction.

carbamazepine	May increase citalopram clearance.	• Monitor patient for clinical effects.
alcohol CNS drugs	May cause additive CNS effects.	• Use together cautiously. Monitor patient for increased sedation, dizziness, agitation, and asthenia. • Advise patient to avoid alcohol.
drugs that inhibit cytochrome P-450 isoenzymes 3A4 and 2C19	May decrease clearance of citalopram.	• Monitor patient for signs of toxicity, including dizziness, sweating, nausea, vomiting, tremor, increased sedation, altered mental status, and ECG changes.
imipramine TCAs	Level of imipramine metabolite desipramine may increase by 50%.	• Monitor patient for adverse effects.
lithium	May enhance serotonergic effect of citalopram.	• Use together cautiously. • Monitor lithium level. • Dosage adjustment may be needed.
MAO inhibitors	Serious, sometimes fatal, reactions may occur.	• Don't use drug within 14 days of MAO inhibitor therapy.
warfarin	Prothrombin time may increase by 5%.	• Monitor PT and INR carefully. • Monitor patient for signs of bleeding.
St. John's wort **sumatriptan**	May increase risk of serotonin syndrome (altered mental status; increased muscle tone, weakness, twitching; hyperthermia; delirium; coma; death).	• Strongly advise against concurrent use of this drug and St. John's wort. • Advise patient to contact a health care professional before using herbal preparations. • Switching from citalopram to St. John's wort requires a wash-out period to eliminate drug from the body.

Interacting agents in **bold type** indicate severe, well-documented interactions.   †Canadian

INTERACTING AGENTS	POSSIBLE EFFECTS	NURSING CONSIDERATIONS
clarithromycin • Biaxin		
cyclosporine phenytoin triazolam	May decrease metabolism of these drugs.	• Monitor patient for toxicity depending on the drug (increased sedation, nausea, vomiting, ataxia, nystagmus, tremor, hyperreflexia, confusion, seizures). • Monitor serum drug levels if appropriate.
digoxin	May increase serum digoxin level.	• Monitor serum digoxin level. • Check for signs of digoxin toxicity.
dihydroergotamine ergotamine	May cause acute ergot toxicity.	• Monitor patient for peripheral ischemia and vasospasm. • Ergot dosage may need to be changed.
carbamazepine theophylline	May increase serum levels of these drugs.	• Monitor theophylline level. • Dosage adjustment may be needed. • Don't use carbamazepine and antibiotics together. Monitor carbamazepine serum levels and monitor patient for toxicity.
warfarin	May increase anticoagulant effect.	• Monitor PT and INR closely. • Monitor patient for signs of bleeding.
pimozide	May increase pimozide level and cardiotoxicity.	• Don't use together. • Monitor ECG and vital signs.
clemastine fumarate • Tavist, Tavist Allergy		
MAO inhibitors	May prolong and intensify the central depressant and anticholinergic effects.	• Avoid using together.
alcohol CNS depressants	May increase sedation.	• Monitor patient for increased adverse effects, including increased sedation, dizziness, agitation, asthenia, and respiratory

| | depression. |
| | • Advise patient to avoid alcohol. |

sulfonylureas	May diminish the effects.	• Monitor serum glucose level. Check for signs of hyperglycemia (fatigue, polyuria, polydipsia, weight loss, abdominal pain, altered mental status, tachycardia, hypotension, glucosuria, ketonuria).
		• Dosage adjustment may be needed.
heparin	May partially counteract the anticoagulant effect.	• Monitor patient for clinical effects.
		• Monitor PTT.
sun exposure	Photosensitivity reactions may occur.	• Advise patient to take precautions.

clonazepam • Klonopin, Rivotril†

alcohol anticonvulsants CNS depressants	May cause additive CNS-depressant effects.	• Monitor patient for increased CNS depression (increased sedation, dizziness, ataxia, altered mental status).
		• Advise patient to avoid alcohol.
valproic acid	May increase sedation and loss of seizure control.	• Monitor patient for loss of clinical effect and increased sedation.
ritonavir	May significantly increase clonazepam level.	• Don't use together, if possible.
		• If used together, monitor patient for sedation and respiratory depression.

clonidine hydrochloride • Catapres, Catapres-TTS, Dixarit†

| alcohol barbiturates | Clonidine may increase CNS-depressant effects of these agents. | • Use together cautiously. Monitor patient for increased sedation, dizziness, agitation, and asthenia. |
| | | • Advise patient to avoid alcohol. |

(continued)

INTERACTING AGENTS	POSSIBLE EFFECTS	NURSING CONSIDERATIONS
clonidine hydrochloride *(continued)*		
MAO inhibitors tolazoline **TCAs**	May inhibit the antihypertensive effects of clonidine.	• Don't use with TCAs. • Monitor BP for clinical effect.
propranolol or other beta blockers	May have an additive effect, producing bradycardia. Severe hypertension may occur if one of these drugs is stopped.	• Consider additive effects. • If drug change is warranted, gradually stop beta blocker first and monitor BP.
yohimbe	May precipitate clonidine withdrawal hypertensive crisis.	• Strongly discourage concomitant use.
clopidogrel bisulfate • Plavix		
aspirin NSAIDs	May increase risk of GI bleeding.	• Use together cautiously. • Monitor patient for increased GI complaints, abdominal pain, and melena.
heparin warfarin	Safety hasn't been established.	• Use together cautiously. • Monitor CBC, PT, PTT, and INR, as appropriate.
red clover	May cause increased bleeding.	• Advise patient to avoid using together. • Advise patient to consult health care provider before taking herbal preparations.
clozapine • Clozaril		
antihypertensives	May potentiate the hypotensive effects.	• Check BP frequently.
anticholinergics	May potentiate the anticholinergic effects of clozapine.	• Avoid using together, if possible.

benzodiazepines	May pose risk of respiratory arrest and severe hypotension.	• Avoid using together. • Discontinue benzodiazepine dose ≥ 1 wk before initiating clozapine.
bone marrow suppressants	May increase bone marrow toxicity.	• Avoid using together, if possible. • Monitor patient for increased bleeding, bruising, and infection. • Monitor hematologic laboratory studies.
alcohol CNS-active drugs	May potentiate additive effects.	• Monitor patient for increased adverse effects, including increased sedation, dizziness, agitation, asthenia, and respiratory depression. • Advise patient to avoid alcohol.
phenytoin	Clozapine may decrease phenytoin level. May lower the seizure threshold.	• Avoid using together, if possible. • Monitor serum phenytoin levels. • Monitor patient for loss of seizure control.
digoxin highly protein-bound drugs (e.g., ritonavir) warfarin	May increase serum levels.	• Monitor serum drug levels. • Monitor patient for clinical effects and drug toxicity.
nutmeg	May reduce effectiveness of drug.	• Advise patient to avoid using together. • Advise patient to consult health care provider before taking herbal preparations.
caffeine	May inhibit antipsychotic effects of clozapine.	• Advise patient to decrease caffeine intake.
smoking	May reduce plasma clozapine level.	• Discourage smoking.

INTERACTING AGENTS	POSSIBLE EFFECTS	NURSING CONSIDERATIONS
colchicine		
cyclosporine	May increase GI toxicity.	• Dose may require adjustment.
erythromycin	May increase serum colchicine level.	• May need to reduce colchicine dosage.
loop diuretics	May decrease efficacy of colchicine prophylaxis.	• Monitor patient for clinical effect.
phenylbutazone	May increase risk of leukopenia or thrombocytopenia.	• Monitor hematologic tests. • Don't use together, if possible.
vitamin B	May impair vitamin absorption	• Monitor patient for vitamin deficiency.
alcohol	May inhibit drug action.	• Advise patient to avoid alcohol.
co-trimoxazole (trimethoprim-sulfamethoxazole) • Apo-Sulfatrim†, Bactrim, Bactrim DS, Bactrim I.V., Cotrim, Cotrim D.S., Novo-Trimel†, Roubact†, Septra, Septra DS, Septra I.V., SMZ-TMP, Sulfatrim		
oral anticoagulants	Co-trimoxazole may inhibit hepatic metabolism, enhancing anticoagulant effects.	• Monitor PT and INR. • Observe patient for signs of bleeding.
PABA	May antagonize sulfonamide effects.	• Monitor patient closely for lack of therapeutic effect.
oral sulfonylureas	May enhance hypoglycemic effects.	• Monitor serum glucose level. • Monitor patient for signs of excessive hypoglycemia (dizziness, diaphoresis, confusion, tachycardia).
phenytoin	Co-trimoxazole may inhibit metabolism of phenytoin.	• Monitor phenytoin levels. • Dosage adjustment may be needed.
TCAs	May decrease antidepressant effect.	• Monitor patient for lack of therapeutic effect.

indomethacin	May increase plasma level of sulfamethoxazole.	• Dosage adjustment may be needed.
digoxin	May increase serum digoxin levels, especially in geriatric patients.	• Monitor serum digoxin level. • Monitor patient for toxicity.
pyrimethamine	May cause megaloblastic anemia in pyrimethamine doses > 25 mg/wk.	• Closely monitor hematologic tests.
methotrexate	May increase methotrexate level.	• Use together cautiously. • Monitor serum methotrexate level.
zidovudine	May increase serum level of zidovudine.	• Monitor patient for adverse effects and toxicity.
cyclosporine	May decrease therapeutic effect and increase risk of nephrotoxicity.	• Don't use together, if possible. • Monitor renal function.
sun exposure	Photosensitivity reaction may occur.	• Advise patient to use sunblock.

cyclizine hydrochloride • Marezine
cyclizine lactate • Marezine, Marzine†

aminoglycosides cisplatin loop diuretics salicylates vancomycin	May mask signs of ototoxicity.	• Avoid this combination, if possible. • Perform a baseline hearing test and monitor periodically thereafter. • Dose reduction or withdrawal of one of the drugs may be needed. • Advise patient of this potential interaction.
alcohol CNS depressants (such as antianxiety drugs, barbiturates, sleeping aids, tranquilizers)	May cause additive sedative and CNS-depressant effects.	• Monitor patient for increased adverse effects, including increased sedation, dizziness, agitation, asthenia, and respiratory depression.

INTERACTING AGENTS	POSSIBLE EFFECTS	NURSING CONSIDERATIONS
cyclobenzaprine hydrochloride • Flexeril		
depressants	May potentiate CNS depression.	• Monitor patient for signs of increased CNS depression, including sedation, dizziness, ataxia, altered mental status, and respiratory depression.
antidyskinetics antimuscarinics	May potentiate antimuscarinic effects.	• Monitor patient for signs of anticholinergic toxicity.
guanadrel guanethidine	Cyclobenzaprine may decrease or block the antihypertensive effects.	• Closely monitor BP.
MAO inhibitors	Hyperpyretic crisis, seizures, and death have occurred from concurrent use of MAO inhibitors and tricyclics; the potential for this interaction with cyclobenzaprine also exists.	• Allow 14 days after stopping MAO inhibitor therapy before starting cyclobenzaprine, and allow 5 to 7 days after stopping cyclobenzaprine therapy before starting MAO inhibitor.
cyclophosphamide • Cytoxan, Neosar		
barbiturates	May increase pharmacologic effects and potentiate toxicity from the increased conversion of cyclophosphamide to active metabolites.	• Use together cautiously. • Monitor patient for signs of severe toxicity, including severe leukopenia and thrombocytopenia, increased GI complaints, and cardiotoxicity.
corticosteroids	May inhibit cyclophosphamide metabolism, reducing its effect.	• Reducing dose or stopping corticosteroid may increase cyclophosphamide to a toxic level. • Use with extreme caution.
allopurinol chloramphenicol chloroquine	May inhibit cyclophosphamide metabolism.	• Monitor patient closely for signs of severe toxicity, including severe leukopenia and thrombocytopenia, increased GI

imipramine phenothiazines potassium iodide vitamin A		complaints, and cardiotoxicity.
succinylcholine	May prolong respiratory distress and apnea.	• Use succinylcholine with caution, if at all.
doxorubicin	Use of cyclophosphamide may potentiate the cardiotoxic effects.	• Monitor cardiac function closely.
digoxin	May decrease serum digoxin level.	• Monitor serum digoxin level and patient for clinical effects; dosage may need adjustment.

cyclosporine • Neoral, Sandimmune

aminoglycosides amphotericin B	May increase nephrotoxicity; amphotericin may increase cyclosporine blood level.	• Don't use together, if possible. • Cyclosporine may need to be reduced during therapy. • Alternative immunosuppressive therapy may be used. • Monitor renal function.
immunosuppressants (except corticosteroids)	May increase risk of malignancy (lymphoma) and susceptibility to infection.	• Don't use together.
azole antifungal drugs corticosteroids **diltiazem** **erythromycin** verapamil	May increase plasma cyclosporine level.	• Monitor cyclosporine and serum creatinine levels. • Reduced dosage of cyclosporine may be needed.
co-trimoxazole **hydantoins** phenobarbital **rifampin**	May lower plasma level of cyclosporine.	• Don't use together, if possible. • If used together, monitor cyclosporine levels and renal function. • Adjust cyclosporine dose as needed.

(continued)

Interacting agents in **bold type** indicate severe, well-documented interactions.   †Canadian

INTERACTING AGENTS	POSSIBLE EFFECTS	NURSING CONSIDERATIONS
cyclosporine *(continued)*		
high-fat diet grapefruit or grapefruit juice	May increase trough blood levels of cyclosporine.	• Don't give with grapefruit or grapefruit juice, or a high-fat meal.
pill-bearing spurge	May inhibit CYP5A enzyme, affecting drug metabolism.	• Discourage concomitant use.
digoxin	May elevate digoxin level with potential toxicity.	• Monitor serum digoxin levels. • Monitor patient for signs of toxicity.
dacarbazine (DTIC) • DTIC-Dome		
anticoagulants aspirin	May increase risk of bleeding.	• Use together cautiously. • Monitor patient for increased bleeding tendencies.
bone marrow suppressants	May cause additive toxicity.	• Monitor hematologic studies. • Monitor patient for increased bleeding, bruising, and infection.
amphotericin B	May increase risk of nephrotoxicity.	• Monitor renal function closely.
phenobarbital phenytoin	May increase risk of toxicity.	• Monitor patient for signs of dacarbazine toxicity, including severe myelosuppression, nausea, vomiting, diarrhea, and abdominal pain.
sun exposure	Photosensitivity reactions may occur, especially during the first 2 days.	• Advise patient to take precautions.
danazol • Cyclomen†, Danocrine		
cyclosporine	May increase cyclosporine level and chance of nephrotoxicity.	• Monitor renal function studies and cyclosporine level.

warfarin-type anticoagulants	May prolong PT and INR.	• Avoid using together, if possible. • Monitor PT and INR. • Dosage adjustment may be needed.
carbamazepine	May increase plasma level of carbamazepine.	• Avoid using together, if possible. • Monitor carbamazepine level. • Monitor patient for signs of toxicity.

delavirdine mesylate • Rescriptor

amphetamines benzodiazepines calcium channel blockers clarithromycin dapsone ergot alkaloid preparations indinavir nonsedating antihistamines quinidine rifabutin saquinavir sedative hypnotics sildenafil warfarin	May increase or prolong therapeutic and adverse effects of these drugs. Delavirdine has an inhibitory effect on the liver enzymes CY3PA and CYP2C9, which metabolize these drugs; there may be increased plasma levels.	• Don't use together, if possible. • Dosage adjustment may be needed. • Monitor patient for adverse effects or signs of toxicity.
clarithromycin fluoxetine ketoconazole	May cause up to a 50% increase in delavirdine trough level.	• Monitor patient closely for increased adverse effects.
carbamazepine phenobarbital phenytoin rifabutin rifampin	May cause a substantial decrease in plasma delavirdine level.	• Coadministration is not recommended.

(continued)

INTERACTING AGENTS	POSSIBLE EFFECTS	NURSING CONSIDERATIONS
delavirdine mesylate (continued)		
antacids	May reduce absorption of delavirdine.	• Give at least 1 hr apart.
H₂-receptor antagonists	May increase gastric pH, which reduces absorption of delavirdine.	• Long-term, concurrent use isn't recommended.
didanosine	May result in 20% decrease in absorption of both drugs.	• Give at least 1 hr apart.
indinavir	May increase plasma level.	• A lower dose of indinavir may be needed.
saquinavir	May cause five-fold increase in saquinavir bioavailability. May increase or prolong therapeutic and adverse effects of these drugs. Delavirdine has an inhibitory effect on the liver enzymes CY3PA and CYP2C9, which metabolize these drugs; there may be increased plasma levels.	• Don't use together, if possible. • If concomitant use is needed, make appropriate dosage adjustments. • Monitor patient for adverse effects or signs of toxicities. • Frequently monitor AST and ALT levels.
demeclocycline hydrochloride • Declomycin		
antacids containing aluminum, calcium, or magnesium laxatives containing aluminum, magnesium, or calcium antidiarrheals food, milk, other dairy products **iron products** sodium bicarbonate zinc	May impair oral absorption of demeclocycline.	• Separate administration times of these agents by 3 to 4 hr. • Enteric-coated or sustained-release iron preparations may be given with tetracycline. • Demeclocycline should be given 1 hr before or 2 hr after food, including dairy products.
digoxin	May increase digoxin level.	• Monitor digoxin level. • Monitor patient for signs of digoxin

		toxicity, including fatigue, asthenia, dizziness, arrhythmias, visual disturbances, nausea, vomiting, and diarrhea. • Dose adjustment may be needed.
methoxyflurane	May increase risk of nephrotoxicity.	• Avoid using together.
oral contraceptives	May decrease contraceptive effect. Breakthrough bleeding has been reported.	• Advise patient to use barrier contraception.
penicillin	May inhibit cell growth from bacteriostatic action.	• Avoid giving these together. • If unavoidable, administer penicillin 2 to 3 hr before tetracycline. • Monitor patient for expected clinical effects.
anticoagulants	May enhance anticoagulation effects.	• Monitor PT and INR. • Dose adjustment may be needed.
sun exposure	Enhances photosensitivity reactions.	• Advise patient to take precautions.

desipramine hydrochloride • Norpramin

beta blockers cimetidine fluoxetine fluvoxamine methylphenidate oral contraceptives paroxetine propoxyphene sertraline	May increase serum desipramine level.	• Monitor patient for desipramine toxicity, including excessive anticholinergic activity followed by increased CNS-depressant effects.
MAO inhibitors	May cause severe excitation, hyperpyrexia, or seizures, usually with high dosage.	• Don't administer desipramine with or within 2 wk of MAO inhibitor therapy.

(continued)

INTERACTING AGENTS	POSSIBLE EFFECTS	NURSING CONSIDERATIONS
desipramine hydrochloride *(continued)*		
ephedrine epinephrine norepinephrine phenylephrine	May increase BP.	• Monitor BP frequently. • Monitor patient for severe hypertension.
warfarin	May increase PT and cause bleeding.	• Monitor PT and INR. • Monitor patient for increased bleeding tendencies.
antiarrhythmics pimozide thyroid hormones	May increase incidence of cardiac arrhythmias and conduction defects.	• Monitor ECG closely when concurrent drug therapy starts.
clonidine guanabenz guanadrel **guanethidine** methyldopa reserpine	Desipramine may decrease hypotensive effects of these drugs.	• Avoid using with clonidine. • When used with other drugs, monitor BP frequently, especially at start of therapy. • Alternative antihypertensive may be needed.
alcohol CNS depressants	May cause additive effects.	• Use together cautiously. • Monitor patient for increased sedation, dizziness, agitation, asthenia, and respiratory depression. • Advise patient to avoid alcohol.
disulfiram ethchlorvynol	May cause delirium and tachycardia.	• Observe patient closely for these adverse effects or other signs of psychosis.
barbiturates	May induce desipramine metabolism and decrease therapeutic efficacy.	• Monitor patient for clinical effect. • Check for increased sedation or respiratory depression. • Dosage adjustment may be needed.

haloperidol phenothiazines	May decrease desipramine metabolism, leading to increased serum levels.	• Monitor serum desipramine level. • Monitor patient for signs of toxicity. • Dosage adjustment may be needed.
quinolones	May cause life-threatening cardiac arrhythmias.	• Don't use together.
SSRIs	May cause desipramine toxicity at much lower dosages.	• Monitor patient for toxicity. • Dosage reduction may be needed.
evening primrose oil	May have an additive or synergistic effect, resulting in a lower seizure threshold and increased risk of seizure.	• Advise patient not to use together. • Advise patient to contact a health care professional before using herbal preparations.
smoking (heavy)	May lower plasma level of desipramine.	• Discourage smoking.
sun exposure	May increase risk of photosensitivity.	• Advise patient to use sunblock.

desmopressin acetate • DDAVP, Stimate

chlorpropamide clofibrate fludrocortisone urea	May potentiate the antidiuretic action of desmopressin.	• Use together cautiously. • Monitor patient for clinical effects and increased adverse effects.
alcohol carbamazepine demeclocycline epinephrine heparin lithium norepinephrine	May decrease the antidiuretic effect.	• Use together cautiously. • Monitor patient for a potential decrease in clinical response. • Advise patient to avoid alcohol.

INTERACTING AGENTS	POSSIBLE EFFECTS	NURSING CONSIDERATIONS
dexamethasone (systemic) • Decadron, Deronil†, Dexasone†, Dexone, Hexadrol **dexamethasone acetate** • Dalalone D.P., Decadron-LA, Decaject-L.A., Dexasone-L.A., Dexone L.A., Solurex LA **dexamethasone sodium phosphate** • AK-Dex, Dalalone, Decadrol, Decadron, Decaject, Dexameth, Dexasone, Dexone, Hexadrol Phosphate, Oradexon†, Solurex		
insulin oral antidiabetics	May cause hyperglycemia.	• Monitor serum glucose level. • Monitor patient for signs of hyper- glycemia. • May require dosage adjustment.
oral anticoagulants	May decrease the effects.	• Monitor PT and INR closely.
isoniazid salicylates	Dexamethasone may increase the metabo- lism of isoniazid and salicylates.	• May require dosage adjustment of isoni- azid or salicylates.
amphotericin B diuretics	May cause hypokalemia.	• Monitor serum potassium level. • Monitor patient for signs of hy- pokalemia, including muscle weakness, fatigue, and arrhythmias.
cardiac glycosides	Hypokalemia may increase the risk of toxi- city.	• Monitor potassium and digoxin levels. • Monitor patient for toxicity.
barbiturates phenytoin **rifampin**	May decrease corticosteroid effects.	• Avoid using together, if possible. • Check for loss of therapeutic effects. • Corticosteroid dosage may need to be increased.
antacids cholestyramine colestipol	May decrease the corticosteroid effects.	• Separate administration times. • Monitor patient closely. • Dosage adjustment may be needed.

estrogens	May reduce the metabolism of dexamethasone by increasing the level of transcortin.	• Dosage adjustment may be needed
alcohol aspirin NSAIDs	May increase the risk of GI ulceration.	• Monitor patient closely for occult bleeding. • Advise patient to avoid alcohol.
toxoids vaccines	May decrease antibody response and increase risk of neurologic complications.	• Vaccine shouldn't be administered during dexamethasone therapy.

dextromethorphan hydrobromide • Balminil D.M.†, Benylin DM Cough, Broncho-Grippol-DM†, Delsym, DM Cough Syrup†, Hold, Koffex†, Mediquell, Neo-DM†, Robidex†, Sedatuss†, St. Joseph Cough Suppressant for Children, Sucrets Cough Control Formula, Suppress, Trocal, Vicks Formula 44

| MAO inhibitors
parsley
selegiline
sibutramine | May cause serotonin syndrome (altered mental status; increased muscle tone, weakness, twitching; hyperthermia; delirium; coma; death). | • Don't use together. Dextromethorphan shouldn't be given to patient who has taken an MAO inhibitor within 2 wk.
• Advise patient against using herbs. |

diazepam • Apo-Diazepam†, Dizac, Novodipam†, Valium, Vivol†, Diastat, Zetran

| alcohol
antidepressants
antihistamines
barbiturates
general anesthetics
MAO inhibitors
narcotics
phenothiazines | Diazepam may potentiate the CNS-depressant effects of these agents. | • Use together cautiously.
• Monitor patient for signs of increased CNS depression, including sedation, dizziness, agitation, asthenia, altered level of consciousness, and increased respiratory depression.
• Advise patient to avoid alcohol. |

(continued)

Interacting agents in **bold type** indicate severe, well-documented interactions.   †Canadian

INTERACTING AGENTS	POSSIBLE EFFECTS	NURSING CONSIDERATIONS
diazepam *(continued)*		
cimetidine disulfiram oral contraceptives	May diminish hepatic metabolism of diazepam, which increases its plasma level.	• Monitor patient closely for increased sedation and impaired judgment. • Diazepam dose may need to be decreased
antacids	May decrease the rate of absorption of diazepam.	• Give at least 2 hr apart.
haloperidol	May change the seizure patterns. May reduce the serum level of haloperidol.	• Monitor patient's seizure activity. • Dosage adjustment may be needed.
digoxin	Diazepam may decrease digoxin clearance.	• Monitor serum digoxin level. • Monitor patient for digoxin toxicity.
nondepolarizing neuromuscular blockers (such as pancuronium and succinylcholine)	May intensify and prolong respiratory depression.	• Monitor patient's vital signs closely.
levodopa	Diazepam may inhibit the therapeutic effect of levodopa.	• Monitor patient for clinical effect.
smoking (heavy)	May accelerate metabolism of diazepam, lowering clinical effectiveness.	• Discourage smoking.
diclofenac potassium • Cataflam **diclofenac sodium** • Voltaren, Voltaren XR		
aspirin	May lower plasma level of diclofenac.	• Avoid using together.
warfarin	May affect platelet function.	• Monitor PT and INR. • Check for increased bleeding tendencies. • Dosage adjustment may be needed.
cyclosporine	May increase the toxicity of these drugs.	• Monitor serum level of appropriate drug.

digoxin methotrexate		• Monitor renal function test results to detect cyclosporine nephrotoxicity. • Monitor patient for signs of digoxin toxicity, including fatigue, asthenia, dizziness, arrhythmias, visual disturbances, nausea, vomiting, and diarrhea. • Monitor patient for signs of methotrexate toxicity, including myelosuppression, anemia, nausea, vomiting, diarrhea, dermatitis, alopecia, melena, and fatigue.
lithium	May decrease renal clearance of lithium and increase plasma level; may lead to lithium toxicity.	• Monitor serum lithium level. • Monitor patient for signs of toxicity, including sedation, confusion, tremors, muscle stiffness, increased deep tendon reflexes, visual changes, and nystagmus.
insulin oral antidiabetics	May alter the patient's response to these drugs.	• Monitor serum glucose level closely. • Monitor patient carefully for signs of hypoglycemia or hyperglycemia. • Dosage adjustment may be needed.
diuretics	Diclofenac may inhibit the action of diuretics.	• Monitor BP and renal function test results.
potassium-sparing diuretics	May increase serum potassium level.	• Monitor serum potassium level closely. • Monitor patient for signs of hyperkalemia, including mental confusion, neuromuscular excitability, weakness, peaked T waves, and widened QRS complex.
beta blockers	May blunt antihypertensive effects.	• Monitor BP.

(continued)

INTERACTING AGENTS	POSSIBLE EFFECTS	NURSING CONSIDERATIONS
diclofenac *(continued)*		
phenytoin	May increase serum level of phenytoin.	• Monitor serum phenytoin level. • Monitor patient for signs of phenytoin toxicity, including drowsiness, confusion or decreased level of consciousness, nausea, vomiting, nystagmus, ataxia, dysarthria, tremor, slurred speech, hypotension, arrhythmias, and respiratory depression.
sun exposure	May cause photosensitivity reactions.	• Advise patient to take precautions.
dicyclomine hydrochloride • Antispas, A-Spas, Bentyl, Bentylol†, Byclomine, Dibent, Formulex†, Lomine†, Neoquess, Or-Tyl, Spasmoban†, Spasmoject		
antacids	May decrease oral absorption of dicyclomine.	• Dicyclomine should be given at least 1 hr before antacids.
amantadine antihistamines antiparkinsonians disopyramide glutethimide meperidine phenothiazines procainamide quinidine TCAs	May cause additive adverse effects related to enhanced anticholinergic activity.	• Monitor patient for signs of toxicity, including mental status changes, hallucinations, xerostomia, visual disturbances, dilated pupils, tachycardia, ECG changes, hyperthermia, hypertension, increased respiratory rate, urinary retention, and constipation. • Dosage adjustments may be needed to avoid toxicity.
ketoconazole levodopa	May decrease GI absorption of these drugs.	• Monitor patient for decreased clinical effect. • Dosage adjustments may be needed.
digoxin (slowly dissolving tablets)	May increase serum digoxin level.	• Closely monitor serum digoxin level. • Monitor patient for digoxin toxicity.

oral potassium supplements (especially wax-matrix formulations)	May increase potassium-induced GI ulcerations.	• Use together cautiously. • Monitor patient for signs of GI ulcerations.
phenothiazines	May decrease therapeutic effect of phenothiazines.	• Monitor patient for clinical effect. • Phenothiazine dose may need to be adjusted.

didanosine (ddl) • Videx, Videx EC

allopurinol	May increase didanosine level.	• Avoid use together.
ganciclovir	May decrease ganciclovir activity.	• Separate administration times by at least 2 hr.
indinavir	May decrease indinavir absorption.	• Give drugs at least 1 hr apart.
dapsone drugs that require gastric acid for adequate absorption itraconazole ketoconazole	May decrease absorption of these drugs from buffers present in didanosine preparations.	• Administer these drugs 2 hr before didanosine.
methadone	May decrease didanosine level.	• Monitor patient closely for clinical effect. • Dosage adjustment may be needed.
fluoroquinolones tetracyclines	May decrease absorption from buffering agents in didanosine tablets or antacids in pediatric suspension.	• Administer tetracyclines at least 2 hr before didanosine. • Administer fluoroquinolones at least 6 hr after didanosine.
antacids containing magnesium or aluminum hydroxide	May produce enhanced adverse effects, such as diarrhea or constipation.	• Be aware that didanosine chewable/dispersable buffered tablets and buffered powder for oral solution already contain agents to increase gastric pH.

(continued)

Interacting agents in **bold type** indicate severe, well-documented interactions.   †Canadian

INTERACTING AGENTS	POSSIBLE EFFECTS	NURSING CONSIDERATIONS
didanosine (ddl) *(continued)*		
		• Unbuffered preparations may be administered with an antacid to increase absorption of the drug.
food	May decrease rate of absorption.	• Give drug on an empty stomach at least 30 min before a meal.
alcohol	May increase risk of pancreatitis.	• Discourage use together.
digoxin • Lanoxicaps, Lanoxin, Novodigoxin†		
amiloride	May inhibit digoxin effect and increase digoxin excretion.	• Monitor for altered digoxin effect.
aminosalicylic acid antacids kaolin-pectin magnesium trisilicate sulfasalazine	May decrease absorption of orally administered digoxin.	• Monitor for altered digoxin effect. • Separate administration times as far as possible.
anticholinergics	May increase digoxin absorption of oral digoxin tablets.	• Monitor serum digoxin level. • Observe patient for toxicity.
cholestyramine colestipol metoclopramide	May impair digoxin absorption.	• Monitor digoxin levels closely. • Give digoxin 1¼ hours before or 2 hours after other drugs.
cytotoxic drugs radiation therapy	May decrease digoxin absorption if the intestinal mucosa is damaged.	• Use of digoxin elixir or capsules is recommended.
amiodarone cyclosporine diltiazem nifedipine	May increase serum digoxin level, predisposing the patient to toxicity.	• Monitor serum digoxin level. • Monitor patient for signs of digoxin toxicity, including fatigue, asthenia, dizziness, arrhythmias, visual disturbances,

oleander **quinidine** squill **verapamil**		nausea, vomiting, and diarrhea. • Advise patient to consult health care provider before using any herbal preparations.
betel palm fumitory goldenseal lily-of-the-valley motherwort procainamide propranolol rue shepherd's purse **verapamil**	May cause additive cardiac effects.	• Monitor patient for increased cardiac effects, including severe bradycardia, hypotension, and arrhythmias. • Advise patient to consult health care provider before using any herbal preparations.
sympathomimetics (such as ephedrine, epinephrine, and isoproterenol, or rauwolfia alkaloids)	May increase risk of arrhythmias.	• Monitor vital signs and ECG closely.
antibiotics	May increase digoxin bioavailability, increasing serum digoxin level.	• Closely monitor serum digoxin level. • Separate administration times.
I.V. calcium	May cause synergistic effects that precipitate arrhythmias.	• Monitor vital signs and ECG closely.
diuretics (such as ethacrynic acid, furosemide, and bumetanide)	May cause hypokalemia and hypomagnesemia.	• Monitor patient's serum electrolyte level closely.
parenteral calcium **thiazide**	May cause hypercalcemia.	• Monitor serum calcium and digoxin levels. • Monitor patient for signs of toxicity.
glucagon large dextrose dose	May elevate digoxin level with potential toxicity.	• Monitor serum digoxin level. • Monitor patient for signs of toxicity.
succinylcholine	May precipitate cardiac arrhythmias by potentiating effects of digoxin.	• Use together cautiously. *(continued)*

Interacting agents in **bold type** indicate severe, well-documented interactions.   †Canadian

INTERACTING AGENTS	POSSIBLE EFFECTS	NURSING CONSIDERATIONS
digoxin (continued)		
amphotericin B carbenicillin corticosteroids corticotropin edetate disodium hawthorn laxatives licorice root sodium polystyrene sulfonate ticarcillin dextrose-insulin infusions	May cause a loss of potassium, predisposing patient to digitalis toxicity.	• Monitor serum potassium and digoxin levels closely.
St. John's wort	May decrease the therapeutic effects of digoxin.	• Strongly discourage concomitant use.
diltiazem hydrochloride • Cardizem, Cardizem CD, Cardizem SR, Dilacor XR, Tiazac		
anesthetics	May increase potential for cardiac depression and vascular dilation.	• Closely monitor vital signs and ECG rhythm.
beta blockers	May combine effects that result in heart failure, conduction disturbances, arrhythmias, and hypotension.	• Use together cautiously. • Monitor patient's vital signs and ECG rhythm.
cyclosporine	May increase serum cyclosporine level and cyclosporine-induced nephrotoxicity.	• Monitor cyclosporine level.
cimetidine	May increase plasma level of diltiazem.	• Monitor patient for toxicity.
digoxin	Diltiazem may increase serum level of digoxin.	• Monitor digoxin level. Monitor patient for toxicity.
carbamazepine	May increase carbamazepine blood level up to 72%.	• Monitor carbamazepine level. • Monitor patient for toxicity.

| theophylline | May increase theophylline level. | • Monitor patient for theophylline toxicity. |

dimenhydrinate • Apo-Dimenhydrinate†, Calm-X, Dimetabs, Dinate, Dommanate, Dramamine, Dramocen, Dramoject, Dymenate, Gravol†, Hydrate, PMS-Dimenhydrinate†, Wehamine

| alcohol
CNS depressants (such as antianxiety drugs, barbiturates, sleeping aids, tranquilizers) | May cause additive CNS sedation and depression. | • Use together cautiously.
• Monitor patient for increased sedation, dizziness, agitation, asthenia, and respiratory depression.
• Advise patient to avoid alcohol. |
| aminoglycosides
cisplatin
loop diuretics
salicylates
vancomycin | Dimenhydrinate may mask the signs of ototoxicity, which can be caused by these drugs. | • Avoid this combination if possible.
• Perform a baseline hearing test and monitor thereafter.
• Advise patient of this interaction. |

diphenhydramine hydrochloride • Benadryl, Benadryl Allergy, Benylin, Compoz, Diphen AF, Diphen Cough, Diphenadryl, Hydramine, Nervine Nighttime Sleep-Aid, Nytol, QuickCaps, Sleep-Eze 3, Sominex, Tusstat, Twilite

MAO inhibitors	May prolong and intensify the central depressant and anticholinergic effects.	• Avoid use together.
alcohol CNS depressants (such as barbiturates, tranquilizers, sleeping aids, antianxiety drugs)	May increase sedation.	• Monitor patient for increased adverse effects, including increased sedation, dizziness, agitation, asthenia, and respiratory depression. • Advise patient to avoid alcohol.
sulfonylureas	Diphenhydramine may diminish the effects of sulfonylureas.	• Monitor serum glucose level. Check for signs of hyperglycemia (fatigue, polyuria, polydipsia, weight loss, abdominal pain, altered mental status, tachycardia, hypotension, glucosuria, ketonuria). • Dosage adjustment may be needed.

(continued)

Interacting agents in **bold type** indicate severe, well-documented interactions.   †Canadian

INTERACTING AGENTS	POSSIBLE EFFECTS	NURSING CONSIDERATIONS
diphenhydramine hydrochloride *(continued)*		
heparin	May partially counteract the anticoagulant effect.	• Monitor patient for clinical effects. • Monitor PTT.
sun exposure	Photosensitivity reactions may occur.	• Advise patient to take precautions.
diphenoxylate hydrochloride and atropine sulfate • Lofene, Logen, Lomanate, Lomotil, Lonox		
MAO inhibitors	May precipitate hypertensive crisis.	• Avoid use together.
alcohol CNS depressants (such as barbiturates, narcotics, tranquilizers)	May increase depressant effect.	• Monitor patient for increased adverse effects, including increased sedation, dizziness, agitation, asthenia, and respiratory depression. • Discourage alcohol use.
dipyridamole • Persantine		
adenosine	May prolong adenosine effects.	• Monitor patient for bradycardia. • Reduce adenosine infusion rate and titrate per response.
aminophylline	May inhibit the coronary vasodilatory action of I.V. dipyridamole.	• Don't use together.
heparin oral anticoagulants	May enhance the effects of oral anticoagulants and heparin.	• Monitor PT, PTT, and INR as indicated. • Monitor patient for increased bleeding tendencies.
disulfiram • Antabuse		
alcohol use (all sources, including cough syrups, liniments, shaving lotions, back-rub preparations)	May precipitate disulfiram reaction.	• Alcohol reaction may occur as long as 2 wk after single disulfiram dose; the longer patient takes drug, the more sensitive he becomes to alcohol.

		• Advise patient to avoid using these products.
barbiturates chlordiazepoxide CNS depressants **coumarin anticoagulants** diazepam midazolam paraldehyde **phenytoin**	Disulfiram may increase the blood levels of these drugs.	• Use together cautiously. • Monitor serum levels. • Monitor patient closely for increased CNS-depressant effects. • Monitor patient for bleeding or bruising tendencies. • Monitor patient for signs of phenytoin toxicity, including drowsiness, confusion, nystagmus, ataxia, arrhythmias, and respiratory depression.
TCAs, especially amitriptyline	May cause transient delirium; tricyclic antidepressant serum level may be increased.	• Monitor patient for signs of acute organic brain syndrome. • Monitor patient for TCA toxicity.
metronidazole	May cause psychosis or confusion.	• Avoid using together.
isoniazid	May cause ataxia, unsteady gait, or marked behavioral changes.	• Don't use together.
caffeine	May exaggerate or prolong effects of caffeine.	• Advise patient to avoid caffeine.
marijuana	Disulfiram may produce synergistic CNS stimulation.	• Inform patient of this interaction.

docetaxel • Taxotere

compounds that induce, inhibit, or are metabolized by cytochrome P-450 3A4 (such as cyclosporine, ketoconazole, erythromycin, troleandomycin)	Docetaxel metabolism may be modified.	• Monitor patient for clinical effects and signs of toxicity, including increased bone marrow suppression, peripheral neurotoxicity, and mucositis.

Interacting agents in **bold type** indicate severe, well-documented interactions.   †Canadian

INTERACTING AGENTS	POSSIBLE EFFECTS	NURSING CONSIDERATIONS
docusate calcium • Pro-Cal-Sof, Surfak **docusate potassium** • Dialose, Diocto-K, Kasof **docusate sodium** • Colace, Diocto, Dioeze, Diosuccin, Disonate, DOK, DOS, Doxinate, D-S-S, Duosol, Modane Soft, Pro-Sof, Regulax SS, Regulex†, Regutol		
mineral oil	Docusate salts may increase absorption of mineral oil and cause toxicity.	• Separate administration times.
dofetilide • Tikosyn		
amiloride amiodarone diltiazem macrolide antibiotics metformin	May increase plasma dofetilide level.	• Use together cautiously, if at all. • Obtain a careful medication history, including herbal and OTC drugs, before giving dofetilide. • Monitor patient for increased adverse effects, including prolonged QT interval and arrhythmias.
class I, class III antiarrhythmics nefazodone norfloxacin protease inhibitors quinine serotonin reuptake inhibitors triamterene zafirlukast	Effect hasn't been studied.	• Concurrent use isn't recommended. • Hold antiarrhythmics for at least three half-lives before giving dofetilide.
drugs that prolong QT interval (bepridil, oral macrolides, phenothiazines, TCAs)	May enhance QT interval prolongation.	• Avoid using together, if possible. • If used together for any reason, closely monitor ECG, especially QT interval.
potassium-wasting diuretics	May increase risk of torsades de pointes.	• Monitor potassium level. • Maintain potassium level within normal range before and during drug therapy.

drugs that inhibit renal cation transport system (cimetidine, ketoconazole, megestrol, prochlorperazine, sulfamethoxazole, trimethoprim) grapefruit juice verapamil	May decrease dofetilide metabolism and excretion and increase plasma level.	• Use with any of these drugs is contraindicated. • Don't give dofetilide with grapefruit juice.

dolasetron mesylate • Anzemet

drugs that prolong ECG intervals (such as antiarrhythmics)	May increase the risk of arrhythmias.	• Monitor patient closely. • Monitor QT interval and ECG for arrhythmias.
drugs that inhibit the P-450 enzymes (such as cimetidine)	May increase hydrodolasetron level.	• Monitor patient for adverse effects, including headache, hypotension, dizziness, bradycardia or tachycardia, dyspepsia, and diarrhea.
drugs that induce the P-450 enzyme (such as rifampin)	May decrease hydrodolasetron level.	• Monitor patient for decreased efficacy of dolasetron mesylate.

donepezil hydrochloride • Aricept

anticholinergics	May interfere with anticholinergic activity.	• Check patient for expected clinical effects.
carbamazepine dexamethasone phenobarbital phenytoin rifampin	May increase rate of elimination of donepezil.	• Monitor patient for clinical effect.
bethanechol cholinesterase inhibitors cholinomimetics jaborandi tree pill-bearing spurge succinylcholine	May produce synergistic effect.	• Monitor patient closely for adverse effects and toxicity. • Discourage concomitant use.

Interacting agents in **bold type** indicate severe, well-documented interactions.   †Canadian

INTERACTING AGENTS	POSSIBLE EFFECTS	NURSING CONSIDERATIONS
dorzolamide hydrochloride • Trusopt		
oral carbonic anhydrase inhibitors	May cause additive effects.	▪ Don't use together.
other ocular hypotensives (betaxolol, carteolol, levobunolol, metipranolol, timolol)	May cause additive IOP-lowering effects.	▪ This combination may be used for therapeutic advantage. ▪ Give drugs at least 10 min apart.
doxazosin mesylate • Cardura		
clonidine	May decrease antihypertensive effects of clonidine.	▪ Monitor BP.
butcher's broom	May reduce effects of doxazosin.	▪ Discourage concomitant use.
doxepin hydrochloride • Adapin, Sinequan, Triadapin†		
beta blockers cimetidine fluoxetine fluvoxamine methylphenidate oral contraceptives paroxetine propoxyphene sertraline	May inhibit doxepin metabolism, increasing plasma level and toxicity.	▪ Monitor patient for signs of doxepin toxicity, including excessive anticholinergic activity followed by increased CNS-depressant effects.
MAO inhibitors	May cause severe excitation, hyperpyrexia, or seizures, usually with high dosage.	▪ Don't administer doxepin with or within 2 wk of MAO inhibitor therapy.
sympathomimetics (such as ephedrine, epinephrine, norepinephrine, phenylephrine)	May increase BP.	▪ Check BP frequently. ▪ Monitor patient for severe hypertension.
warfarin	May increase PT and cause bleeding.	▪ Monitor PT and INR. ▪ Look for signs of increased bleeding.

antiarrhythmics (such as disopyramide, procainamide, quinidine) pimozide thyroid hormones	May increase incidence of cardiac arrhythmias and conduction defects.	• Monitor ECG closely when concurrent drug therapy starts.
centrally acting antihypertensive drugs (such as **clonidine**, guanabenz, guanadrel, guanethidine, methyldopa, reserpine)	Doxepin may decrease hypotensive effects.	• Don't use with clonidine. • When used with other drugs, monitor BP frequently, especially when therapy starts. • Alternative antihypertensive may be needed.
alcohol CNS depressants	May have additive effects.	• Use together cautiously. • Monitor patient for increased sedation, dizziness, agitation, asthenia, and respiratory depression. • Advise patient to avoid alcohol.
disulfiram ethchlorvynol	May cause delirium and tachycardia.	• Observe patient closely for these adverse effects and other signs of psychosis.
anticholinergics atropine	May cause oversedation, paralytic ileus, visual changes, and severe constipation.	• Use these drugs together only when needed. • Monitor patient for increased sedation, respiratory depression and GI or visual complaints. • Dosage adjustment may be needed.
metrizamide	May increase risk of seizures.	• Monitor patient closely for increased seizures.
barbiturates	May induce doxepin metabolism and decrease therapeutic efficacy.	• Monitor patient for clinical effect and increased sedation or respiratory depression. • Dosage adjustment may be needed.

(continued)

INTERACTING AGENTS	POSSIBLE EFFECTS	NURSING CONSIDERATIONS
doxepin hydrochloride (continued)		
haloperidol phenothiazines	May decrease metabolism of doxepin, leading to increased serum levels.	• Monitor serum doxepin level. • Monitor patient for signs of toxicity. • Dosage adjustment may be needed.
quinolones	May potentiate life-threatening cardiac arrhythmias.	• Don't use together.
SSRIs	Patient may become toxic to doxepin at much lower dosage.	• Monitor patient for toxicity. • Dosage reduction may be needed.
evening primrose oil	May have additive or synergistic effect, resulting in lower seizure threshold and increased risk of seizure.	• Advise patient not to use together. • Advise patient to contact a health care professional before using herbal preparations.
smoking (heavy)	May lower plasma levels of doxepin.	• Discourage smoking.
sun exposure	May increase risk of photosensitivity.	• Advise patient to wear sunblock.
doxycycline • Vibramycin		
antacids containing aluminum, calcium, or magnesium laxatives containing magnesium oral iron products sodium bicarbonate zinc	May decrease oral absorption of doxycycline.	• Give doxycycline 1 hr before or 2 hr after these agents.
alcohol carbamazepine phenobarbital	May decrease doxycycline effect.	• Doxycycline dose may be increased or another tetracycline may be chosen. • Advise patient to avoid alcohol.

digoxin	May increase bioavailability of digoxin.	• Monitor serum digoxin level. • Digoxin dosage may be lowered.
methoxyflurane	May cause nephrotoxicity.	• Don't use together.
oral anticoagulants	May increase anticoagulant effect.	• Monitor PT and INR. • Dosage adjustment may be needed.
oral contraceptives	May decrease contraceptive effectiveness and increase risk of breakthrough bleeding.	• Advise patient to use barrier contraception.
penicillin	May antagonize bactericidal effects.	• Don't use together.
sun exposure	May cause photosensitivity reactions.	• Advise patient to use sunblock.
econazole • Ecostatin†, Spectazole		
corticosteroids	May inhibit the antifungal activity of econazole nitrate, in a level-dependent manner, in the treatment of *Saccharomyces* and *Candida albicans*.	• Avoid using together.
edrophonium chloride • Enlon, Reversol, Tensilon		
aminoglycosides anesthetics	May enhance neuromuscular blockade.	• Use together cautiously.
cardiac glycosides	May increase the heart's sensitivity to edrophonium.	• Monitor vital signs and ECG.

(continued)

INTERACTING AGENTS	POSSIBLE EFFECTS	NURSING CONSIDERATIONS
edrophonium chloride *(continued)*		
cholinergics	May lead to additive toxicity.	• Avoid using together. • If used together, monitor patient for toxicity symptoms, including muscle weakness, nausea, vomiting, diarrhea, miosis, bronchospasm, hypotension, excessive sweating, paralysis, bradycardia, or tachycardia.
corticosteroids	May decrease the cholinergic effects of edrophonium; when corticosteroids are stopped, however, cholinergic effects may increase, possibly affecting muscle strength.	• Observe patient for lack of drug effect. • Profound muscular weakness may occur in patients with myasthenia gravis; monitor patient closely.
ganglionic blockers (such as mecamylamine)	May lead to a critical BP decrease.	• Avoid using together. If used together, monitor BP and other vital signs closely.
magnesium	May cause a direct depressant effect on skeletal muscle. May antagonize therapeutic effects of edrophonium chloride.	• Avoid using together, if possible.
procainamide quinidine	May reverse the cholinergic effect of edrophonium on muscle.	• Avoid using together, if possible.
succinylcholine	May prolong respiratory depression from plasma esterase inhibition.	• Use this combination cautiously. • Monitor respirations, other vital signs, and the return of spontaneous muscle activity.
jaborandi tree pill-bearing spurge	May cause an additive effect and increase risk of toxicity.	• Advise patient against using together. • Advise patient to contact a health care

professional before using an herbal preparation.

efavirenz • Sustiva

ergot derivatives midazolam triazolam	Competition for cytochrome P-450 enzyme system may inhibit the metabolism of these drugs and cause serious or life-threatening adverse events (such as arrhythmias, prolonged sedation, or respiratory depression).	• Don't administer together.
clarithromycin indinavir	May decrease plasma levels of these drugs.	• Alternative therapy or dosage adjustment may be needed.
drugs that induce the cytochrome P-450 enzyme system (such as phenobarbital, rifampin, rifabutin)	May increase clearance of efavirenz, resulting in a lower plasma level.	• Monitor patient closely for expected clinical effects.
estrogens ritonavir	May increase plasma levels of these drugs; ritonavir also increases efavirenz level.	• Monitor patient for increased adverse effects.
oral contraceptives	Interaction of efavirenz with oral contraceptives hasn't been determined.	• Advise patient to also use a reliable method of barrier contraception.
alcohol psychoactive drugs	May cause additive CNS effects.	• Monitor patient for increased sedation, dizziness, agitation, and asthenia. • Advise patient to avoid alcohol.
saquinavir	Decreases plasma level of saquinavir significantly.	• Don't use with saquinavir as sole protease inhibitor.
warfarin	May increase or decrease plasma level and effects of warfarin.	• Avoid using together, if possible. • If used together, monitor PT and INR.

(continued)

Interacting agents in **bold type** indicate severe, well-documented interactions.   †Canadian

INTERACTING AGENTS	POSSIBLE EFFECTS	NURSING CONSIDERATIONS
efavirenz (continued)		
St. John's wort	May decrease efavirenz level.	• Advise patient against using together. • Advise patient to contact a health care professional before using an herbal preparation.
high-fat meals	May increase absorption of efavirenz.	• Instruct patient to maintain a low-fat diet.
enalaprilat • Vasotec I.V. **enalapril maleate** • Vasotec		
antihypertensives diuretics phenothiazines	May increase antihypertensive effects.	• Use together cautiously. • Dosage adjustments may be needed. • Diuretic dose may need to be decreased or the drug stopped.
insulin oral antidiabetics	May increase risk of hypoglycemia, especially when enalapril therapy starts.	• Monitor serum glucose level. • Observe patient for signs of excessive hypoglycemia (dizziness, diaphoresis, confusion, tachycardia).
lithium	May decrease renal clearance of lithium.	• Monitor lithium level. • Monitor patient for signs of toxicity.
aspirin NSAIDs	May decrease the antihypertensive effect of enalapril.	• Avoid using together, if possible. • If used together, monitor BP.
potassium-sparing diuretics potassium supplements	May enhance diuretic effects and possibly hyperkalemia.	• Monitor renal function and serum potassium level. • Monitor patient for signs of hyperkalemia.

rifampin	May decrease pharmacologic effects of rifampin.	• Monitor patient for clinical effect.
salt substitutes	May enhance effects, causing hyperkalemia.	• Caution patient to avoid salt substitutes.

enoxaparin sodium • Lovenox

anticoagulants antiplatelets NSAIDs	May increase risk of bleeding. May also lead to spinal or epidural hematomas in patients with spinal punctures or epidural or spinal anesthesia.	• Discontinue these drugs before using enoxaparin unless absolutely necessary. • If used together, monitor patient for increased bleeding tendencies. • Monitor CBC and coagulation studies. • Check stool for occult blood.
plicamycin valproic acid	May cause hypoprothrombinemia and inhibit platelet aggregation.	• Monitor patient closely for increased bleeding. Monitor coagulation effects.

entacapone • Comtan

ampicillin chloramphenicol cholestyramine erythromycin probenecid	May block biliary excretion, resulting in higher serum level of entacapone.	• Monitor patient for increased adverse effects, including dyskinesia, hyperkinesia, dizziness, nausea, diarrhea, abdominal pain, and urine discoloration.
alcohol CNS depressants	May have an additive effect.	• Should be used together cautiously. • Monitor patient for increased sedation, dizziness, agitation, and asthenia. • Advise patient to avoid alcohol.
drugs metabolized by COMT (bitolterol, dobutamine, dopamine, epinephrine, isoetharine, isoproterenol, norepinephrine)	May cause higher serum levels of these drugs, resulting in increased HR, changes in BP or, possibly, arrhythmias.	• Use together very cautiously. • Monitor patient's vital signs and ECG.

(continued)

INTERACTING AGENTS	POSSIBLE EFFECTS	NURSING CONSIDERATIONS
entacapone *(continued)*		
nonselective MAO inhibitors (such as phenelzine, tranylcypromine)	May inhibit normal catecholamine metabolism.	• Avoid using together.
ephedrine • ephedrine hydrochloride • ephedrine sulfate • Pretz-D		
acetazolamide	May increase serum ephedrine level.	• Monitor patient for toxicity.
alpha-adrenergic blockers	May reduce vasopressor response, resulting in hypotension.	• Monitor BP. • Monitor patient for expected effects.
antihypertensives	May decrease effects of antihypertensives.	• Monitor BP.
atropine	May block reflex bradycardia and enhance pressor effects.	• Monitor HR and BP.
beta blockers	May block cardiac and bronchodilating effects of ephedrine.	• Monitor BP. • Monitor patient for adverse effects.
ergot alkaloids	May enhance vasoconstrictor activity.	• Monitor patient for tachycardia, arrhythmias, hypertension, and headache.
cardiac glycosides general anesthetics (especially cyclopropane, halothane)	May sensitize myocardium to effects of ephedrine, causing arrhythmias.	• Avoid using together, if possible. • If used together, monitor vital signs and ECG for arrhythmias.
guanadrel guanethidine	May enhance pressor effects of ephedrine.	• Monitor patient closely. • Monitor BP.
levodopa	May enhance risk of ventricular arrhythmias.	• If used together, monitor ECG closely for arrhythmias.
MAO inhibitors TCAs	May enhance pressor effects; may cause hypertensive crisis.	• Allow 14 days to lapse after withdrawal of MAO inhibitor before using ephedrine. • If used with a TCA, monitor patient for arrhythmias and hypertension.

		• Dosage adjustment may be needed.
diuretics methyldopa reserpine	May decrease pressor effects of ephedrine.	• Monitor patient for expected response.
sympathomimetics	May increase effects and toxicity.	• Avoid using together.
theophylline	May cause more adverse reactions than either drug when used alone.	• Monitor patient for increased adverse effects.

epinephrine • Bronkaid Mist, Bronkaid Mistometer†, EpiPen, EpiPen Jr., Primatene Mist, Sus-Phrine
epinephrine bitartrate • AsthmaHaler
epinephrine hydrochloride • Adrenalin Chloride, AsthmaNefrin, Epifrin, Glaucon, microNefrin, Vaponefrin
epinephryl borate • Epinal

sympathomimetics	May increase effects and toxicity.	• Avoid using together.
alpha blockers	May antagonize vasoconstriction and hypertension.	• Monitor BP. • Monitor patient closely for expected clinical effects.
antidiabetics	May decrease serum glucose effects.	• Monitor serum glucose level. • Dosage adjustments may be needed.
beta blockers (such as propranolol)	May increase BP with reflex bradycardia.	• Avoid using together. • Beta blocker should be discontinued 3 days before anticipated epinephrine use. • Monitor BP. • Monitor patient for adverse respiratory effects.
doxapram mazindol methylphenidate	May enhance CNS stimulation or pressor effects.	• Monitor patient for increased adverse effects, such as hypertension, tachycardia, arrhythmias, restlessness, anxiety, tremors, headache, and insomnia.

(continued)

INTERACTING AGENTS	POSSIBLE EFFECTS	NURSING CONSIDERATIONS
epinephrine *(continued)*		
general anesthetics (especially cyclopropane, **halothane**) cardiac glycosides	May sensitize the myocardium to effects of epinephrine, causing arrhythmias.	• Don't use together.
guanadrel guanethidine	May decrease hypotensive effects while potentiating effects of epinephrine, resulting in hypertension and arrhythmias	• Monitor patient closely. • Monitor BP.
levodopa	May enhance risk of cardiac arrhythmias.	• Monitor ECG closely for arrhythmias.
MAO inhibitors	May increase risk of hypertensive crisis.	• Monitor BP closely.
miotics	May reduce ciliary spasm, mydriasis, and blurred vision, and may increase intraocular pressure that can occur with miotics or epinephrine alone.	• May be used together for this clinical effect.
oxytocics ergot alkaloids	May cause severe hypertension.	• Monitor patient for tachycardia, arrhythmias, hypertension, and headache.
phenothiazines	May reverse pressor effects.	• Avoid using together, if possible. • Monitor patient for clinical effects.
antihistamines thyroid hormones TCAs	May potentiate adverse cardiac effects of epinephrine.	• Monitor vital signs and ECG closely.
epirubicin hydrochloride • Ellence		
calcium channel blockers cardioactive compounds	May increase risk of heart failure.	• Monitor cardiac function closely.
cimetidine	May increase epirubicin level by 50%.	• Avoid using together.

| cytotoxic drugs | May cause additive toxicities (especially hematologic and gastrointestinal). | • Monitor patient for increased GI complaints, such as vomiting.
• Monitor hematologic studies. |
| radiation therapy | May increase cardiotoxic effects of radiation in the mediastinal or pericardial area. | • If possible, don't give drug during radiation therapy; an inflammatory recall reaction may occur at the radiation site. |

eptifibatide • Integrilin

| dipyridamole
NSAIDs
oral anticoagulants
thrombolytics
ticlopidine | May increase risk of bleeding. | • Monitor patient for increased bleeding or bruising tendencies.
• Monitor hematologic and coagulation studies and stool for occult blood. |
| inhibitors of platelet receptor GP IIb/IIIa | May potentiate serious bleeding. | • Don't give together. |

ergotamine tartrate • Cafergot, Ergomar, Ergostat, Gynergen, Medihaler Ergotamine, Wigraine

erythromycin macrolides	May cause symptoms of ergot toxicity evidenced by peripheral ischemia.	• Monitor patient for symptoms of ergot toxicity. Vasodilators (nifedipine, nitroprusside, or prazosin) may be ordered to treat ergot toxicity.
propranolol or other beta blockers	May increase vasoconstrictor effects.	• Monitor patient for peripheral ischemia.
protease Inhibitors	May cause symptoms of ergot toxicity evidenced by peripheral vasospasm and ischemia of the extremities.	• Avoid using together.
selective 5-HT1 receptor agonists (naratriptan, rizatriptan, sumatriptan, zolmitriptan)	May prolong vasospastic reactions.	• Don't give ergotamine within 24 hr of giving these drugs.

(continued)

INTERACTING AGENTS	POSSIBLE EFFECTS	NURSING CONSIDERATIONS
ergotamine tartrate *(continued)*		
sibutramine	May potentiate serotonin syndrome (altered mental status, increased muscle tone, weakness, twitching; hyperthermia; delirium; coma; death).	• Avoid using together.
caffeine	May increase rate and extent of absorption.	• Advise patient to avoid caffeine.
alcohol	May worsen headaches.	• Advise patient to avoid alcohol.
smoking	May increase adverse effects.	• Discourage smoking.
erythromycin • E-Base, E-Mycin, ERYC, Ery-Tab, Ilotycin, PCE, Robimycin		
carbamazepine	May increase carbemazepine blood level and increase risk of toxicity.	• Carbamazepine should not be given with erythromycin. • If drugs are given together, carbamazepine serum level must be monitored. Monitor the patient for toxicity.
clindamycin lincomycin	May cause antagonistic bactericidal activity.	• Don't use together.
cyclosporine	May increase serum cyclosporine level and nephrotoxicity.	• Monitor cyclosporine and serum creatinine levels. Reduced dosage of cyclosporine may be needed.
digoxin	May increase serum digoxin level.	• Monitor patient for digitalis toxicity.
disopyramide quinolones	May increase disopyramide plasma level, possibly causing arrhythmias and increased QT intervals.	• Monitor ECG.
isotretinoin	May cause cumulative dryness, resulting	• Monitor patient's skin integrity.

in excessive skin irritation.

midazolam triazolam	May increase effects of these drugs.	• Monitor patient for increased sedation.
oral anticoagulants	May have excessive anticoagulant effect.	• Monitor PT and INR closely when starting or stopping erythromycin therapy.
theophylline	May increase serum theophylline level and decrease erythromycin blood level.	• Monitor serum theophylline level. • Monitor erythromycin's clinical effect. • Consider an alternative anti-infective drug.
pill-bearing spurge	May inhibit CYP3A enzymes, affecting drug metabolism.	• Discourage use together.
soaps or cleansers (abrasive or medicated) acne preparations or preparations containing peeling agents (benzoyl peroxide, resorcinol, salicylic acid, sulfur, tretinoin) alcohol-containing products (aftershave, perfumed toiletries, cosmetics, shaving creams or lotions) astringent soaps or cosmetics medicated cosmetics or cover-ups	May cause cumulative dryness, resulting in excessive dryness.	• Monitor patient's skin integrity. • Advise patient to consult health care provider before using OTC preparations. • Patient should wash, rinse, and dry skin thoroughly before using a topical erythromycin preparation.

esmolol hydrochloride • Brevibloc

insulin oral antidiabetics	May mask symptoms of developing hypoglycemia.	• Monitor serum glucose level. • Drug may mask signs of excessive hypoglycemia (dizziness, diaphoresis, confusion, tachycardia).
antihypertensives	May potentiate their hypotensive effects.	• Monitor BP. • Dosage adjustments may be needed.

(continued)

INTERACTING AGENTS	POSSIBLE EFFECTS	NURSING CONSIDERATIONS
esmolol hydrochloride (continued)		
digoxin (I.V.)	May increase digoxin blood level by 10% to 20%.	• Monitor serum digoxin level. • Dosage adjustment may be needed.
morphine (I.V.)	May increase esmolol steady-state level by 50%.	• Monitor patient carefully. • Titrate esmolol dose gradually.
nondepolarizing neuromuscular blockers (such as succinylcholine, gallamine, metocurine, pancuronium, or tubocurarine)	May potentiate and prolong their action.	• Carefully monitor patient postoperatively after concurrent or sequential use, especially if there's a possibility of incomplete reversal of neuromuscular blockade.
catecholamine-depleting drugs reserpine	May cause additive and possibly excessive beta-adrenergic blockade with bradycardia and hypotension.	• Monitor vital signs closely. • Monitor patient for complaints of dizziness or syncope.
sympathomimetic amines with beta-adrenergic–stimulant activity	May cause mutual but transient inhibition of therapeutic effects.	• Use together cautiously. • Monitor patient for clinical effect.
xanthines, especially aminophylline or theophylline	May cause mutual inhibition of therapeutic effects and (except for dyphylline) may decrease theophylline clearance, especially in patients with increased theophylline clearance induced by smoking.	• Monitor patient carefully to prevent toxic accumulation of theophylline.
verapamil	May cause additive effects.	• Avoid using together, if possible. • If used together, monitor cardiac function. • Dosage adjustments may be needed.
clonidine	May cause potentially life-threatening hypertension.	• Monitor BP closely when these drugs are used together and after one is discontinued.

estazolam • ProSom

disulfiram isoniazid oral contraceptives	May diminish hepatic metabolism, resulting in increased plasma level of estazolam.	• Monitor patient for increased sedation. • Estazolam dose may need to be decreased or dosing interval extended.
alcohol antihistamines barbiturates general anesthetics MAO inhibitors narcotics phenothiazines TCAs	May increase CNS effects.	• Monitor patient closely for increased sedation or other signs of CNS depression. • Dosage decrease may be needed. • Advise patient to avoid alcohol.
digoxin phenytoin	May increase levels of these drugs and cause toxicity.	• Monitor serum digoxin or phenobarbital levels. • Monitor patient for signs of toxicity.
probenecid	May increase benzodiazepine effect.	• Monitor patient for increased effects of estazolam, especially increased sedation and lethargy. • Dosage adjustment may be needed.
rifampin	May increase clearance and decrease half-life of estazolam.	• Monitor patient for decreased drug effect.
theophylline	May antagonize pharmacologic effects of estazolam.	• Monitor patient for expected clinical effect.
smoking (heavy)	May accelerate metabolism of estazolam, resulting in diminished clinical efficacy.	• Discourage smoking.
caffeine	May enhance CNS effects.	• Discourage use together.

Interacting agents in **bold type** indicate severe, well-documented interactions.   †Canadian

INTERACTING AGENTS	POSSIBLE EFFECTS	NURSING CONSIDERATIONS
estradiol • Climara, Estrace, Vivelle		
drugs that induce hepatic metabolism (such as rifampin, barbiturates, primidone, carbamazepine, phenytoin)	May decrease estrogenic effects from a given dose.	• Monitor patient for clinical effect. Menstrual irregularities and breakthrough bleeding may occur. Advise patient to use barrier contraception. • Monitor patient for seizure control.
insulin oral antidiabetics	May increase serum glucose level.	• Monitor serum glucose level. • Antidiabetic dosage may need adjustment.
warfarin-type anticoagulants	May decrease anticoagulant effect.	• Monitor PT and INR. • Anticoagulant dose may need adjustment.
corticosteroids	May cause enhanced corticosteroid effects.	• Monitor patient for clinical and toxic effects of corticosteroids.
cyclosporine	May increase risk of cyclosporine toxicity.	• Monitor patient and cyclosprine level frequently.
dantrolene hepatotoxic drugs	May increase risk of hepatotoxicity.	• Monitor serum liver enzymes. • Monitor patient for liver toxicity.
tamoxifen	May decrease effects of tamoxifen.	• Monitor patient closely for expected clinical effects of tamoxifen.
caffeine	May increase serum caffeine level.	• Advise patient to avoid caffeine.
smoking	May increase risk of adverse CV effects.	• Discourage smoking.
estrogen and progestin • Alesse-28, Brevicon, Demulen 1/35, Demulen 1/35-28, Enovid, Loestrin 21 1/20, Loestrin 21 1.5/30, Loestrin Fe 1/20, Loestrin Fe 1.5/30, Lo/Ovral, Lo/Ovral-28, Modicon 21, Modicon 28, Nordette-21, Nordette-28, Norinyl 1+35 21-Day, Norinyl 1+35 28-Day, Norinyl 1+50 21-Day, Norinyl 1+50 28-Day, Norinyl 1+80 28-Day, Ortho-Novum 1/35 21, Ortho-Novum 1/35 28, Ortho-Novum 1/50 21, Ortho-Novum 1/50 28, Ortho-Novum 7/7/7-21, Ortho-Novum 7/7/7-28, Ortho-Novum 10/11-21, Ortho-Novum 10/11-28, Ovcon-35, Ovcon-50, Ovral, Ovral-28, Tri-Norinyl-21, Tri-Norinyl-28, Triphasil-21, Triphasil-28		
aminoglutethimide	May increase metabolism of oral contra-	• Monitor patient for clinical effects

ampicillin antihistamines barbiturates carbamazepine chloramphenicol griseofulvin isoniazid neomycin nitrofurantoin penicillin V phenylbutazone phenytoin primidone rifampin sulfonamides tetracycline	ceptives, resulting in reduced efficacy, breakthrough bleeding, and, occasionally, contraceptive failure.	• Instruct patient to inform health care provider of adverse effects, such as menstrual irregularities or breakthrough bleeding. • Advise patient of the potential for contraceptive failure when using an estrogen/progesterone combination with these drugs. • Advise patient to use barrier contraception when using these drugs for a short time. • Advise patient to consider other forms of birth control if more prolonged therapy is needed.
insulin oral antidiabetics	May increase serum glucose level.	• Monitor serum glucose level. • Antidiabetic dosage may need adjustment.
oral warfarin-type anticoagulants anticonvulsants antihypertensives TCAs	Countereffects of these drugs may occur.	• Monitor patient for clinical effects of appropriate agent. • Monitor PT, INR, and BP. • Monitor patient for loss of seizure control. • Monitor patient for antidepressant effects. • Monitor patient for TCA toxicity.
caffeine	May increase serum caffeine level.	• Advise patient to avoid caffeine.
smoking	May increase risk of CV effects.	• Discourage smoking.

Interacting agents in **bold type** indicate severe, well-documented interactions.   †Canadian

INTERACTING AGENTS	POSSIBLE EFFECTS	NURSING CONSIDERATIONS
etodolac • Lodine, Lodine XL		
antacids	May decrease peak levels of the drug.	• Monitor patient for decreased effects of etodolac. • Separate administration times by 2 hr.
aspirin	May reduce protein-binding of etodolac without altering its clearance and may increase GI toxicity.	• Monitor patient for clinical effects. • Monitor patient for adverse GI effects.
cyclosporine	May impair elimination and increase risk of nephrotoxicity.	• Monitor cyclosporine level and renal function test results.
digoxin lithium methotrexate	May increase levels of these drugs.	• Monitor serum drug levels. • Monitor patient for signs of drug toxicity.
diuretics beta blockers	May blunt effects of these drugs.	• Monitor patient for fluid retention and BP control. • Adjust dose p.r.n.
phenytoin	May increase serum level of phenytoin.	• Monitor patient for signs of toxicity.
warfarin	May decrease protein-binding of warfarin but doesn't change its clearance.	• Monitor PT and INR and watch for bleeding. • No dosage adjustment is needed.
alcohol	May increase risk of adverse effects.	• Advise patient to avoid alcohol.
sun exposure	Photosensitivity reactions may result.	• Advise patient to take precautions.
etoposide • Toposar, VePesid		
cisplatin	Etoposide may increase cytotoxicity of cisplatin against certain tumors.	• May be used for this clinical effect.

| warfarin | May prolong PT and INR. | • Monitor patient for increased bleeding or bruising tendencies.
• Monitor PT and INR. |
| cyclosporine | May elevate etoposide serum level. | • Monitor CBC.
• Monitor patient for toxicity. |

exemestane • Aromasin

| CYP3A4 inducers | May decrease exemestane plasma level. | • Monitor patient closely for expected clinical effects. |
| estrogens | May inactivate exemestane. | • Avoid using together. |

famciclovir • Famvir

| probenecid | May increase plasma level of penciclovir, the active metabolite of famciclovir. | • Monitor patient for increased adverse effects. |

famotidine • Pepcid, Pepcid AC

| enteric-coated drugs | Enteric coatings may dissolve too rapidly because of increased gastric pH. | • Separate administration times. |
| ketoconazole | May decrease absorption of ketoconazole. | • Ketoconazole dose may need to be increased. |

felodipine • Plendil

anticonvulsants	May decrease plasma level of felodipine.	• Monitor patient for clinical effect. • Patient may need a higher felodipine dosage.
cimetidine	May decrease clearance of felodipine.	• Use lower doses of felodipine.
digoxin	May decrease peak serum level of digoxin, but total absorbed drug is unchanged.	• Clinical significance is unknown. • Monitor patient's serum digoxin level.

(continued)

Interacting agents in **bold type** indicate severe, well-documented interactions.   †Canadian

INTERACTING AGENTS	POSSIBLE EFFECTS	NURSING CONSIDERATIONS
felodipine (continued)		
metoprolol	May alter the pharmacokinetics of metoprolol.	• Monitor patient for adverse effects. • No dosage adjustment is needed.
theophylline	May slightly decrease theophylline level.	• Monitor patient for clinical drug effects. • Monitor theophylline serum level.
grapefruit juice	May increase bioavailability and effect of drug.	• Don't use together.
fenofibrate (micronized) • Tricor		
coumarin-type anticoagulants	May cause protein-binding displacement of the anticoagulant and potentiation of its effects.	• Avoid this combination, if possible. • If used together, use extreme caution. • Reduce dose of anticoagulant to maintain PT and INR within desired range.
HMG-CoA inhibitors (statins)	No data are available on use of statins with fenofibrate, but the use of statins with gemfibrozil (another fibrate derivative) may cause myopathy, rhabdomyolysis, and acute renal failure.	• Avoid using together, if possible. • If used together, monitor patient for signs of myopathy and rhabdomyolysis (increased serum creatinine kinase level, muscle aches, weakness).
bile acid resins	May bind and inhibit absorption of fenofibrate.	• Fenofibrate should be taken 1 hr before or 4 to 6 hr after taking these drugs.
cyclosporine	Cyclosporine-induced renal dysfunction may compromise the elimination of fenofibrate.	• Use together cautiously. • Monitor renal function; monitor patient for increased adverse effects.
fenoldopam mesylate • Corlopam		
beta blockers	Beta-blocker inhibition of the reflex response to fenoldopam may cause unexpected hypotension.	• Avoid using together, if possible. • If used together, monitor BP closely.

fentanyl transdermal system • Duragesic-25, Duragesic-50, Duragesic-75, Duragesic-100

CNS depressants general anesthetics hypnotics MAO inhibitors narcotic analgesics sedatives TCAs alcohol	May cause additive CNS-depressant effects.	• Use together cautiously. • Monitor patient closely for increased CNS depressant effects (sedation, dizziness, ataxia, tremor, agitation, respiratory depression). • Doses of fentanyl and other agent may need to be reduced. • Advise patient to avoid alcohol.
diazepam	May cause CV depression when given with high doses of fentanyl.	• Monitor vital signs and ECG closely.
droperidol	May cause hypotension and decreased pulmonary arterial pressure.	• Monitor vital signs and hemodynamic function closely.
amiodarone	May cause bradycardia, sinus arrest, and hypotension.	• Monitor vital signs and ECG closely.

ferrous sulfate • Apo-Ferrous Sulfate†, Feosol, Feratab, Fer-In-Sol, Fer-Iron, Fero-Grad-500†, Fero-Gradumet, Ferospace, Ferralyn Lanacaps, Ferra-TD, Mol-Iron, Novoferrosulfat†, PMS Ferrous Sulfate†, Slow FE

antacids aluminum-containing phosphate binder cholestyramine cimetidine vitamin E	May decrease iron absorption.	• Separate doses by 1- to 2-hr intervals.
chloramphenicol	May delay response to iron therapy from bone marrow suppression.	• If possible, use an alternative antibiotic. • If used together, monitor iron level. • Dosage adjustment may be needed.

(continued)

INTERACTING AGENTS	POSSIBLE EFFECTS	NURSING CONSIDERATIONS
ferrous sulfate *(continued)*		
doxycycline	May interfere with iron absorption even when doses are separated.	• Separate administration times by 3 to 4 hr to minimize effect. • May use an enteric-coated or sustained-release iron preparation.
L-thyroxine	May decrease L-thyroxine absorption.	• Separate doses by at least 2 hr. • Monitor thyroid function.
levodopa methyldopa	May decrease absorption of these drugs.	• Separate administration times. • Monitor patient for clinical response.
penicillamine	May decrease penicillamine absorption.	• Separate doses by at least 2 hr.
quinolones	Drug may decrease absorption of quinolones from formation of an iron-quinolone complex.	• Separate administration times.
tetracycline	May inhibit absorption of both drugs.	• Give tetracycline 3 hr after or 2 hr before iron supplement.
vitamin C	May increase iron absorption.	• May be used as a beneficial effect.
cheese cereals coffee eggs milk tea whole-grain breads yogurt	May impair oral iron absorption.	• Avoid giving iron preparations with these foods or beverages.

finasteride • Propecia, Proscar

theophylline	May cause clinically insignificant increases in theophylline clearance and decreased half-life (10%).	• Monitor serum theophylline level.

flecainide acetate • Tambocor

acidifying and alkalinizing drugs	Alkalinization may decrease renal flecainide excretion, and acidification may increase it.	• Monitor patient carefully for expected clinical response and signs of increased adverse reactions and toxicity. • Dosage adjustment may be needed.
amiodarone drugs that inhibit P450 IID6 (quinidine, ritonavir)	May increase plasma level of flecainide.	• Monitor serum drug level. • Monitor patient for signs of toxicity, such as prolonged PR and QT intervals, increased QRS complex duration, heart failure, and hypotension. • Flecainide dose may need to be decreased.
beta blockers	May cause additive negative inotropic effects.	• Monitor vital signs and ECG.
digoxin	May increase serum digoxin level.	• Monitor digoxin level. • Monitor patient for signs of digoxin toxicity, including fatigue, asthenia, dizziness, arrhythmias, visual disturbances, nausea, vomiting, and diarrhea.
cimetidine	May decrease both the renal and nonrenal clearance of flecainide.	• Monitor patient for toxicity.

(continued)

INTERACTING AGENTS	POSSIBLE EFFECTS	NURSING CONSIDERATIONS
flecainide acetate (continued)		
carbonic anhydrase inhibitors high-dose antacids sodium bicarbonate	May have a marked effect on urine acidity.	• Monitor patient for possible subtherapeutic or toxic levels and effects.
disopyramide verapamil	These drugs have negative inotropic effects.	• Don't administer these drugs with flecainide unless the risks outweigh the benefits.
smoking	May lower flecainide serum level.	• Discourage smoking.
fluconazole • Diflucan		
cimetidine	May reduce serum level of fluconazole.	• Monitor patient for clinical effects.
cyclosporine	May increase cyclosporine level.	• Monitor cyclosporine level and renal function test results.
hydrochlorothiazide	May decrease fluconazole clearance, elevating serum level of the drug.	• Monitor patient for increased adverse effects (headache, GI disturbances, hepatotoxicity).
phenytoin	May significantly increase serum phenytoin level.	• Monitor serum phenytoin level.
rifampin	May decrease fluconazole level.	• Monitor patient for clinical effects.
isoniazid phenytoin rifampin sulfonylureas valproic acid	May elevate hepatic transaminase level.	• Monitor liver function test results. • Monitor patient for signs of hepatotoxicity (jaundice, fever, abdominal pain, clay-colored stools, tea-colored urine).
glipizide glyburide	May increase hypoglycemic effects.	• Observe patient for signs of excessive hypoglycemia (dizziness, diaphoresis,

		confusion, tachycardia).
sulfonylureas tolbutamide		
tacrolimus	May increase tacrolimus level.	• Monitor renal function and tacrolimus level. • Dosage adjustment may be needed.
theophylline	May increase theophylline level.	• Monitor theophylline level.
warfarin	May enhance hypoprothrombinemic effects.	• Monitor PT and INR closely.
zidovudine	May increase activity of zidovudine.	• Monitor patient for adverse effects.
caffeine	May increase plasma caffeine level.	• Advise patient to avoid caffeine.
vinca alkaloids (vinblastine, vincristine)	May increase risk of vinca alkaloid toxicity.	• Don't use together, if possible. • If used together, monitor patient for vinca alkaloid toxicity.

flumazenil • Romazicon

antidepressants drugs that can cause seizures or arrhythmias	May cause seizures or arrhythmias after flumazenil removes the effects of the benzodiazepine overdose.	• Flumazenil shouldn't be used in mixed overdose, especially when seizures (from any cause) are likely to occur.
food	Ingestion of food during an I.V. infusion of flumazenil may increase drug clearance by 50%.	• Observe patient for lack of clinical effect.

fluoxetine • Prozac, Prozac Pulvules

cyproheptadine	May reverse or decrease pharmacologic effect of fluoxetine.	• Monitor patient for decreased antidepressant effect. Consider stopping cyproheptadine if this occurs.
carbamazepine flecainide vinblastine	May increase serum levels of these drugs.	• Monitor patient for adverse effects.

(continued)

Interacting agents in **bold type** indicate severe, well-documented interactions.   †Canadian

INTERACTING AGENTS	POSSIBLE EFFECTS	NURSING CONSIDERATIONS
fluoxetine *(continued)*		
insulin oral antidiabetics	May alter blood glucose level.	• Monitor serum glucose level. • Dosage adjustment may be needed.
lithium TCAs	May increase adverse CNS effects.	• Monitor TCA or lithium levels as appropriate. Monitor patient for increased sedation, dizziness, agitation, tremor, asthenia, and headache.
phenytoin	May increase serum phenytoin level and risk of toxicity.	• Monitor serum phenytoin level. • Dosage adjustment may be needed.
tryptophan	May increase adverse CNS effects (agitation, restlessness) and GI distress.	• Use together cautiously. • Monitor patient for adverse effects.
highly protein-bound drugs warfarin	May increase plasma levels of fluoxetine or other highly protein-bound drugs.	• Monitor patient for increased adverse effects of these drugs. • Monitor PT and INR if applicable.
MAO inhibitors sibutramine sumatriptan sympathomimetics	May increase risk of serotonin syndrome (altered mental status; increased muscle tone, weakness, twitching; hyperthermia; delirium; coma; death).	• Avoid using with sympathomimetics, sibutramine, or sumatriptan, if possible. • If used together, monitor patient for increased CNS effects. • Don't use with MAO inhibitors. Allow 5 wk or longer between stopping fluoxetine and starting an MAO inhibitor, or 2 wk or longer between stopping the MAO inhibitor and starting fluoxetine.
alcohol	May increase CNS depression.	• Advise patient to avoid alcohol.

fluphenazine decanoate • Modecate†, Prolixin Decanoate
fluphenazine enanthate • Moditen Enanthate†, Prolixin Enanthate
fluphenazine hydrochloride • Permitil, Prolixin

aluminum- and magnesium-containing antacids and antidiarrheals	May inhibit absorption.	• Separate administration times by at least 2 hr.
antiarrhythmics disopyramide procainamide quinidine quinolones (sparfloxacin)	May increase risk of arrhythmias and conduction defects.	• Use together cautiously. • Monitor vital signs and ECG closely. • Don't use sparfloxacin with fluphenazine.
anticholinergics (including antidepressants, MAO inhibitors, phenothiazines, antihistamines, meperidine, and antiparkinsonians) atropine	May cause oversedation, paralytic ileus, visual changes, and severe constipation.	• Use together only when needed. • Monitor patient closely for adverse effects. • Dosage adjustment or discontinuation of therapy may be needed.
beta blockers	May inhibit fluphenazine metabolism, increasing plasma level and toxicity.	• Dosage adjustment may be needed.
bromocriptine	Fluphenazine may antagonize the therapeutic effect of bromocriptine on prolactin secretion.	• Avoid using together. If used together, monitor patient for clinical effect. • Bromocriptine dose may need to be increased.
centrally acting antihypertensives (such as guanethidine, guanabenz, guanadrel, clonidine, methyldopa, reserpine)	May inhibit BP response.	• Monitor BP carefully. • Dosage adjustment or discontinuation of therapy may be needed.

(continued)

INTERACTING AGENTS	POSSIBLE EFFECTS	NURSING CONSIDERATIONS
fluphenazine *(continued)*		
alcohol CNS depressants (including analgesics, barbiturates, narcotics, tranquilizers, and general, spinal, or epidural anesthetics) parenteral magnesium sulfate	May cause additive effects of oversedation, respiratory depression, and hypotension.	• Monitor patient closely for signs of increased CNS depression, including increased sedation, headache, dizziness, ataxia, confusion, agitation, respiratory depression, and hypotension. • Advise patient to avoid alcohol.
dopamine	May decrease vasoconstricting effects.	• Monitor patient closely for clinical response.
levodopa	May decrease effectiveness of levodopa and increase toxicity of levodopa.	• Monitor patient for clinical response to levodopa.
lithium	May result in severe neurologic toxicity with an encephalitis-like syndrome and a decreased therapeutic response to fluphenazine.	• Monitor patient very closely. • Dose may need to be reduced or one or both of the drugs stopped.
metrizamide	May increase risk of seizures.	• Monitor patient closely for increased seizures.
nitrates	May cause hypotension.	• Monitor BP.
phenobarbital	May enhance renal excretion of fluphenazine.	• Dosage adjustment may be needed.
phenytoin TCAs	May inhibit metabolism and increase toxicity of these drugs.	• Monitor serum phenytoin levels. • Check for signs of phenytoin toxicity, including drowsiness, confusion or decreased level of consciousness, nausea, vomiting, nystagmus, ataxia, dysarthria, tremor, slurred speech, hypotension, arrhythmias, and respiratory depression.

		• Monitor patient for signs of TCA toxicity, including excessive anticholinergic activity (agitation, confusion, hallucinations, hyperthermia, seizures, urinary retention, pupillary dilatation, dry mucous membranes) followed by increased CNS depressant effects (decreased or absent reflexes, sedation, respiratory depression, hypotension, arrhythmias, hypothermia). • Dosage adjustment may be needed.
propylthiouracil	May increase risk of agranulocytosis.	• Monitor hematologic studies.
sympathomimetics (including epinephrine, phenylephrine, ephedrine [often in nasal sprays], and appetite suppressants)	May decrease stimulatory and pressor effects; possible epinephrine reversal (hypotensive response to epinephrine).	• Monitor patient for clinical effect. • Tell patient not to take appetite suppressants. • Don't use epinephrine in emergencies, such as severe hypotension; fluphenazine may block the vasopressor effects.
caffeine	May increase metabolism of fluphenazine.	• Advise patient to avoid caffeine.
smoking	May increase metabolism of fluphenazine.	• Discourage smoking.
sun exposure	May increase risk of photosensitivity.	• Tell patient to take precautions.
flurazepam hydrochloride • Apo-Flurazepam†, Dalmane, Novoflupam†		
alcohol antidepressants antihistamines barbiturates general anesthetics MAO inhibitors narcotics phenothiazines	Flurazepam may potentiate the CNS-depressant effects of these agents.	• Monitor patient closely for increased sedation or other signs of CNS depression. • Flurazepam dose may need to be decreased or the dosing interval extended. • Advise patient to avoid alcohol.

(continued)

Interacting agents in **bold type** indicate severe, well-documented interactions.   †Canadian

INTERACTING AGENTS	POSSIBLE EFFECTS	NURSING CONSIDERATIONS
flurazepam (continued)		
digoxin	May increase serum digoxin level.	• Monitor serum digoxin level.
cimetidine disulfiram isoniazid oral contraceptives ritonavir	May decrease metabolism of benzodi- azepines, leading to toxicity.	• Monitor patient for increased sedation. • Flurazepam dose may need to be de- creased or the dosing interval extended.
levodopa	May decrease therapeutic effect of levodopa.	• Monitor patient for clinical effects.
phenytoin	May increase phenytoin level.	• Monitor serum phenytoin level. • Check for signs of phenytoin toxicity, in- cluding drowsiness, confusion, or de- creased level of consciousness; nausea; vomiting; nystagmus; ataxia; dysarthria; tremor; slurred speech; hypotension; ar- rhythmias; and respiratory depression.
rifampin	The effects of flurazepam may decrease with use of rifampin.	• Monitor for clinical effect. • Dosage adjustment may be needed.
theophylline	May act as an antagonist with flurazepam.	• Monitor for clinical effect. • Dosage adjustment may be needed.
catnip kava lady's slipper lemon balm passionflower sassafras skullcap valerian	May enhance sedative effects.	• Discourage patient from using together. • Advise patient to contact a health care provider before using an herbal prepara- tion.

smoking (heavy)	May accelerate metabolism of flurazepam.	• Discourage smoking. • Monitor patient for drug effect.

flurbiprofen • Ansaid

oral anticoagulants	May increase bleeding tendencies.	• Monitor PT and INR. Monitor patient for increased bleeding tendencies. • Dosage adjustment may be needed.
aspirin	May decrease flurbiprofen level and increase GI toxicity.	• Avoid using together, if possible. • Monitor patient for increased GI complaints, abdominal pain, melena, and increased bleeding or bruising tendencies.
beta blockers	May impair antihypertensive effect of beta blockers.	• Monitor BP.
cyclosporine	May increase risk of nephrotoxicity.	• Use together with extreme caution. • Monitor renal function test results.
diuretics	May decrease diuretic effect.	• Monitor renal function test results. • Monitor patient for clinical effect.
lithium	May increase lithium level.	• Monitor serum lithium level. • Monitor patient for signs of toxicity (sedation, confusion, tremors, muscle stiffness, increased deep tendon reflexes, visual changes, nystagmus).
methotrexate	May increase risk of methotrexate toxicity.	• Monitor serum methotrexate level. • Monitor patient for signs of toxicity, including myelosuppression, anemia, nausea, vomiting, diarrhea, dermatitis, alopecia, melena, and fatigue (methotrexate).
alcohol	May increase risk of adverse GI reactions.	• Advise patient to avoid alcohol.

(continued)

INTERACTING AGENTS	POSSIBLE EFFECTS	NURSING CONSIDERATIONS
flurbiprofen • Ansaid		
sun exposure	May potentiate photosensitivity reactions.	• Advise patient to take precautions.
fluvastatin sodium • Lescol		
cholestyramine colestipol	May bind fluvastatin in the GI tract and decrease absorption.	• Administer fluvastatin at bedtime, at least 2 hr after the resin, to avoid significant interaction from the drug binding to the resin.
cimetidine omeprazole ranitidine	May decrease fluvastatin metabolism.	• Monitor patient for decreased drug effect.
cyclosporine erythromycin gemfibrozil immunosuppressants niacin	May increase risk of polymyositis and rhabdomyolysis.	• Don't use together, if possible. • If used together, monitor patient for myolysis and rhabdomyolysis (increased serum creatinine kinase level, muscle aches, weakness).
digoxin	May alter pharmacokinetics of digoxin.	• Monitor patient's serum digoxin level carefully.
rifampin	May enhance fluvastatin metabolism and decrease plasma level.	• Monitor patient closely for lack of effect.
warfarin	May increase anticoagulant effect with bleeding.	• Monitor PT and INR closely. • Monitor patient for increased bleeding tendencies.
alcohol	May increase risk of hepatotoxicity.	• Advise patient to avoid alcohol.
fluvoxamine maleate • Luvox		
benzodiazepines	May reduce clearance of these drugs.	• Use together cautiously. Monitor serum

theophylline warfarin		theophylline level. Monitor PT and INR. • Monitor patient for increased sedation, increased bleeding tendencies, or signs of theophylline toxicity, including tachycardia, nausea, vomiting, diarrhea, restlessness, headaches, agitation, palpitations, and arrhythmias. • Don't give diazepam with fluvoxamine. • Dosage adjustment may be needed.
carbamazepine clozapine methadone metoprolol propranolol TCAs	May elevate serum level of fluvoxamine.	• Use together with caution and monitor patient closely for adverse reactions. • Dosage adjustments may be needed.
diltiazem	May cause bradycardia.	• Monitor patient's HR.
lithium	May enhance effects of fluvoxamine.	• Monitor patient for increased adverse effects, including sedation, dizziness, agitation, tremor, asthenia, headache, nausea, or vomiting.
MAO inhibitors	May cause severe excitation, hyperpyrexia, myoclonus, delirium, and coma.	• Avoid using during or within 2 wk of MAO inhibitor therapy.
sibutramine sumatriptan sympathomimetics	May increase risk of serotonin syndrome (altered mental status; increased muscle tone, weakness, twitching; hyperthermia; delirium; coma; death).	• Don't use fluvoxamine with these drugs, if possible. • If used together, monitor patient for increased CNS effects.
smoking	May decrease effectiveness of drug.	• Discourage smoking.

Interacting agents in **bold type** indicate severe, well-documented interactions.   †Canadian

INTERACTING AGENTS	**POSSIBLE EFFECTS**	**NURSING CONSIDERATIONS**
folic acid • Folvite		
aminosalicylic acid chloramphenicol methotrexate oral contraceptives pyrimethamine sulfasalazine triamterene trimethoprim	These drugs may act as antagonists to folic acid.	• Monitor patient for decreased drug effect. • Monitor folic acid level and CBC for megaloblastic or macrocytic anemia.
anticonvulsants (such as phenobarbital and phenytoin)	May increase anticonvulsant metabolism and decrease blood level of the anticonvulsant.	• Monitor serum blood levels. • Monitor patient for clinical effects.
phenytoin primidone	May decrease serum folate level; symptoms of folic acid deficiency occur in long-term therapy.	• Monitor serum folate level. • Dosage may need adjustment.
pyrimethamine	May interfere with antimicrobial actions of pyrimethamine against toxoplasmosis.	• Don't use together.
foscarnet sodium (phosphonoformic acid) • Foscavir		
nephrotoxic drugs (such as amphotericin B, aminoglycosides, cyclosporine)	May increase risk of nephrotoxicity.	• Avoid using together unless the benefits outweigh the risks. • Monitor renal function test results.
pentamidine (I.V.)	May increase risk of nephrotoxicity; severe hypocalcemia has also been reported.	• Don't use together unless the benefits outweigh the risks.
zidovudine	May increase incidence or severity of anemia.	• Monitor hematologic studies.

fosfomycin tromethamine • Monurol

metoclopramide	May lower serum level and urinary excretion of fosfomycin.	• Avoid using together, if possible. • Monitor patient for increased adverse effects, including headache, dizziness, nausea, diarrhea, and vaginitis.
drugs that increase GI motility	May increase GI effects.	• Monitor patient for these effects.

fosinopril sodium • Monopril

antacids	May impair absorption of fosinopril.	• Separate administration by at least 2 hr.
antihypertensives diuretics	Excessive hypotension may occur.	• Use together cautiously. • Dosage adjustments may be needed. • Diuretic dose may need to be decreased or the drug stopped.
lithium	May increase serum lithium level and lithium toxicity.	• Monitor serum lithium level. • Monitor patient for signs of toxicity, including sedation, confusion, tremors, muscle stiffness, increased deep tendon reflexes, visual changes, and nystagmus.
potassium supplements potassium-sparing diuretics potassium-containing salt substitutes	May result in hyperkalemia.	• Monitor renal function and serum potassium level. Monitor patient for signs of hyperkalemia. • Advise patient to avoid using potassium salt substitutes.

fosphenytoin sodium • Cerebyx

acute alcohol use drugs that may increase plasma phenytoin levels (and thus its therapeutic effects) (such as amiodarone, chloramphenicol, chlordiazepoxide, cimetidine, diazepam,	May increase phenytoin level.	• Monitor phenytoin level. • Check for signs of fosphenytoin toxicity, including drowsiness, confusion or decreased level of consciousness, nausea, *(continued)*

INTERACTING AGENTS	POSSIBLE EFFECTS	NURSING CONSIDERATIONS
fosphenytoin sodium (continued)		
dicumarol, disulfiram, estrogens, etho- suximide, fluoxetine, H₂ antagonists, halothane, isoniazid, methylphenidate, phenothiazines, phenylbutazone, salicy- lates, succinimides, sulfonamides, tolbutamide, trazodone)		vomiting, nystagmus, ataxia, dysarthria, tremor, slurred speech, hypotension, ar- rhythmias, and respiratory depression. • Monitor serum fosphenytoin levels if any of these agents are discontinued while patient is still taking fosphenytoin. • Dosage adjustment may be needed. • Advise patient to avoid alcohol.
carbamazepine reserpine long-term alcohol use	May decrease serum phenytoin level.	• Monitor patient closely for clinical effec- tiveness of fosphenytoin therapy. • Monitor patient for seizure control. • Monitor serum fosphenytoin level. • Dosage adjustments may be needed. • Advise patient to avoid alcohol.
coumarin **cyclosporine** digitoxin doxycycline estrogens furosemide oral contraceptives quinidine rifampin theophylline vitamin D	Phenytoin may decrease efficacy through increased hepatic metabolism.	• Use together cautiously. • Monitor patient for expected clinical ef- fects. • Monitor therapeutic drug levels of these agents if appropriate. • Dosage adjustment may be needed. • If used with oral contraceptives, advise patient to use barrier contraception.
phenobarbital sodium valproate valproic acid	May increase or decrease plasma pheny- toin level.	• Monitor serum fosphenytoin level. • Monitor patient for clinical effect and signs of toxicity.

| TCAs | May lower seizure threshold and may require adjustments in phenytoin dosage. | • Use together cautiously.
• Monitor patient for adequate and previously attained seizure control. |

furosemide • Apo-Furosemide†, Lasix, Lasix Special†, Novosemide†, Uritol†

aminoglycoside antibiotics cisplatin ethacrynic acid	May potentiate ototoxicity.	• Don't use together, if possible. • If used together, obtain baseline hearing test and monitor periodically thereafter. • Dose reduction or withdrawal of one of the drugs may be needed.
antidiabetics	May decrease hypoglycemic effects.	• Monitor serum glucose level. • Check for signs of hyperglycemia (fatigue, polyuria, polydipsia, weight loss, abdominal pain, altered mental status, tachycardia, hypotension, glucosuria, ketonuria). • Dosage adjustment may be needed.
antihypertensives	May increase risk of hypotension.	• Monitor patient's BP frequently.
cardiac glycosides lithium neuromuscular blockers	May increase risk of toxicity of these drugs.	• Monitor serum cardiac glycoside or lithium levels. • Monitor serum potassium level. • Monitor patient for signs of toxicity, including fatigue, asthenia, dizziness, arrhythmias, nausea, vomiting, diarrhea, increased or prolonged respiratory depression and sedation, confusion, tremors, muscle stiffness, increased deep tendon reflexes, visual changes, and nystagmus.
amphotericin B corticosteroids corticotropin	May increase risk of hypokalemia.	• Monitor serum potassium level. • Monitor patient for signs of hypokalemia, including muscle weakness, fa-

(continued)

INTERACTING AGENTS	POSSIBLE EFFECTS	NURSING CONSIDERATIONS
furosemide *(continued)*		
metolazone		tigue, nausea, vomiting, constipation, respiratory depression, and arrhythmias.
NSAIDs	May inhibit diuretic response.	• Monitor patient for clinical response. • Dosage adjustment may be needed.
salicylates	May cause salicylate toxicity.	• Monitor patient for signs of salicylate toxicity, including increased respiratory rate, tinnitus, vomiting, headache, irritability, and seizures.
sucralfate	May reduce diuretic and antihypertensive effect.	• Separate administration by 2 hr.
aloe	May increase drug effects.	• Advise patient to use together cautiously. • Advise patient to consult health care provider before using an herbal preparation.
sun exposure	May potentiate photosensitivity reactions.	• Advise patient to take precautions.
ganciclovir (DHPG) • Cytovene		
cytotoxic drugs	May cause additive toxicity (bone marrow depression, stomatitis, alopecia).	• Use together cautiously. • Monitor patient closely for increased adverse effects. • Monitor hematologic studies.
imipenem-cilastatin	May increase risk of seizures.	• Avoid using together.
immunosuppressants (such as azathioprine, cyclosporine, corticosteroids)	May enhance immune and bone marrow suppression.	• Monitor patient for signs of infection. • Monitor hematologic studies.

nephrotoxic drugs (cyclosporine, amphotericin B)	May increase risk of renal impairment.	• Monitor renal function test results closely.
probenecid	May decrease renal clearance of ganciclovir.	• Monitor patient closely for increased adverse effects.
zidovudine	May increase risk of hematologic toxicity.	• Avoid using together.
sun exposure	May potentiate photosensitivity reactions.	• Advise patient to take precautions.

gatifloxacin • Tequin

antacids containing aluminum or magnesium didanosine buffered tablets, buffered powder, or buffered solution ferrous sulfate zinc, magnesium, or iron products	May decrease absorption of gatifloxacin.	• Give gatifloxacin 4 hr before these products.
antidiabetics (glyburide, insulin)	May cause symptomatic hypoglycemia or hyperglycemia.	• Monitor serum glucose level.
antipsychotics erythromycin TCAs	May prolong QT interval.	• Use cautiously. • Monitor ECG.
class IA antiarrhythmics (quinidine, procainamide), class III antiarrhythmics (amiodarone, sotalol)	May prolong QT interval.	• Avoid using together.
digoxin	May increase digoxin level.	• Monitor serum digoxin level. • Monitor for signs of digoxin toxicity.
NSAIDs	May potentiate increased risk of CNS stimulation and seizures.	• Monitor patient for evidence of seizure activity.

(continued)

INTERACTING AGENTS	POSSIBLE EFFECTS	NURSING CONSIDERATIONS
gatifloxacin (continued)		
probenecid	May increase gatifloxacin level and prolong its half-life.	• May be used together for this effect.
warfarin	May enhance effects of warfarin.	• Monitor PT and INR. • Monitor patient for increased bleeding tendencies.
sun exposure	May cause photosensitivity reactions.	• Advise patient to take precautions.
gemfibrozil • Lopid		
oral anticoagulants	May enhance effect of oral anticoagulants, increasing risk of hemorrhage.	• Monitor PT and INR. • Dosage adjustment may be needed. • Don't use together, if possible. • Monitor for increased bleeding tendencies.
lovastatin pravastatin simvastatin	Myopathy with rhabdomyolysis may occur.	• Monitor patient for signs of myopathy and rhabdomyolysis (increased serum creatinine kinase level, muscle aches, weakness).
gentamicin sulfate • Cidomycin†, G-myticin, Garamycin, Genoptic, Genoptic S.O.P., Gentacidin, Gentak, Gentafair, Gentasol, Jenamicin		
antiemetic and antivertigo drugs dimenhydrinate	May mask gentamicin-induced ototoxicity.	• Advise patient of this potential interaction. • Avoid this combination if possible. • Reduction of dose or withdrawal of one of the drugs may be needed.
bumetanide **ethacrynic acid**	May increase risk of ototoxicity.	• Avoid this combination, if possible.

furosemide mannitol urea		• If used together, obtain a baseline hearing test and monitor periodically thereafter. • Reduction of dose or withdrawal of one of the drugs may be needed.
general anesthetics or neuromuscular blockers (such as succinylcholine and tubocurarine)	May increase neuromuscular blockade.	• Use together only when needed. • Monitor respiratory status and vital signs closely. • Dosage reduction may be needed.
indomethacin (I.V.)	May increase serum peak and trough levels of gentamicin.	• Recommend monitoring serum gentamicin level closely.
acyclovir aminoglycosides amphotericin B capreomycin **cephalosporins** cisplatin methoxyflurane polymyxin B vancomycin	May increase the hazard of nephrotoxicity, ototoxicity, or neurotoxicity.	• Use together cautiously. • Monitor serum drug levels. Monitor renal function test results. • Obtain a baseline hearing test and monitor periodically thereafter. • Monitor patient for increased lethargy, dizziness, confusion, headache, and seizures.
penicillin	May result in synergistic bactericidal effect against *Pseudomonas aeruginosa, Escherichia coli, Enterobacter, Serratia, and Proteus mirabilis*; however, the drugs are physically and chemically incompatible and are inactivated when mixed or given together.	• Don't mix together. Give these drugs at separate times.

(continued)

INTERACTING AGENTS	POSSIBLE EFFECTS	NURSING CONSIDERATIONS
glimepiride • Amaryl		
beta blockers	May mask symptoms of hypoglycemia.	• Monitor serum glucose level closely. • Monitor patient carefully for signs of hypoglycemia, including dizziness, diaphoresis, confusion, and tachycardia.
insulin	May increase potential for hypoglycemia.	• Monitor serum glucose level. • Dosage adjustment may be needed.
NSAIDs drugs that are highly protein-bound (salicylates, sulfonamides, chloramphenicol, coumarins, probenecid, MAO inhibitors, beta blockers)	May potentiate the hypoglycemic action of sulfonylureas, such as glimepiride.	• Monitor serum glucose level closely. • Monitor patient carefully for signs of hypoglycemia, including dizziness, diaphoresis, confusion, and tachycardia. • Dosage adjustment may be needed.
corticosteroids diuretics estrogens isoniazid nicotinic acid oral contraceptives phenothiazines phenytoin sympathomimetics thiazides thyroid hormones	May produce hyperglycemia.	• Monitor serum glucose level closely. • Monitor patient for signs of hyperglycemia (fatigue, polyuria, polydipsia, weight loss, abdominal pain, altered mental status, tachycardia, hypotension, glucosuria, ketonuria). • Dosage adjustment may be needed.
alcohol	May alter glycemic control, most commonly hypoglycemia. May also cause disulfiram-like reaction of nausea, vomiting, abdominal cramps, and headaches.	• Advise patient to avoid alcohol.

adrenocorticoids amphetamines baclofen corticotropin epinephrine estrogens ethacrynic acid furosemide glucocorticoids oral contraceptives phenytoin thiazide diuretics thyroid hormones triamterene	May increase glucose level.	• Monitor serum glucose level. • Monitor patient for signs of hyper-glycemia (fatigue, polyuria, polydipsia, weight loss, abdominal pain, altered mental status, tachycardia, hypotension, glucosuria, ketonuria). • Dosage adjustment may be needed.
anabolic steroids chloramphenicol clofibrate guanethidine insulin MAO inhibitors probenecid salicylates sulfonamides	May enhance hypoglycemic effect by dis-placing glipizide from protein-binding sites.	• Monitor serum glucose level closely. • Monitor patient carefully for signs of hy-poglycemia, including dizziness, di-aphoresis, confusion, and tachycardia. • Dosage adjustment may be needed.
anticoagulants	May increase plasma levels of both drugs and, after continued therapy, may re-duce plasma level and effectiveness of the anticoagulant.	• Monitor serum glucose level and PT and INR. • Dosage adjustment may be needed.

(continued)

Interacting agents in **bold type** indicate severe, well-documented interactions.   †Canadian

INTERACTING AGENTS	POSSIBLE EFFECTS	NURSING CONSIDERATIONS
glipizide *(continued)*		
antifungal antibiotics (such as fluconazole and miconazole)	May increase plasma level of glipizide and cause hypoglycemia.	• Monitor serum glucose level closely. • Monitor patient carefully for signs of hypoglycemia, including dizziness, diaphoresis, confusion, and tachycardia. • Dosage adjustment may be needed.
cimetidine	May potentiate hypoglycemic effects by preventing hepatic metabolism.	• Monitor serum glucose level closely. • Monitor patient carefully for signs of hypoglycemia, including dizziness, diaphoresis, confusion, and tachycardia. • Dosage adjustment may be needed.
beta blockers, including ophthalmics	May mask symptoms of hypoglycemia.	• Monitor patient closely for signs of hypoglycemia, including dizziness, diaphoresis, confusion, and tachycardia. • Dosage adjustment may be needed.
corticosteroids glucagons rifampin thiazide diuretics	May decrease hypoglycemic response.	• Monitor serum glucose level closely. • Monitor patient carefully for signs of hypoglycemia, including dizziness, diaphoresis, confusion, and tachycardia. • Dosage adjustment may be needed.
hydantoins	May increase serum level of hydantoins.	• Monitor serum levels of these drugs.
alcohol	May alter glycemic control. May also cause a disulfiram-like reaction of nausea, vomiting, abdominal cramps, and headaches.	• Advise patient to avoid alcohol.
smoking	May increase corticosteroid release, requiring higher dosages.	• Discourage smoking.

adrenocorticoids amphetamines baclofen corticotropin diazoxide epinephrine ethacrynic acid furosemide glucagons glucocorticoids phenytoin rifampin thiazide diuretics thyroid hormones triamterene	May increase serum glucose level.	• Monitor serum glucose level. • Monitor patient for signs of hyper- glycemia (fatigue, polyuria, polydipsia, weight loss, abdominal pain, altered mental status, tachycardia, hypotension, glucosuria, ketonuria). • Dosage adjustment may be needed.
anabolic steroids chloramphenicol clofibrate guanethidine insulin MAO inhibitors probenecid salicylates sulfonamides	May enhance hypoglycemic effect by dis- placing glyburide from its protein-bind- ing sites.	• Monitor serum glucose level closely. • Monitor patient carefully for signs of hy- poglycemia, including dizziness, di- aphoresis, confusion, and tachycardia. • Dosage adjustment may be needed.
anticoagulants	May increase plasma levels of both drugs and, after continued therapy, may re- duce plasma level and effectiveness of the anticoagulant.	• Monitor serum glucose and PT and INR. • Dosage adjustment may be needed.

(continued)

Interacting agents in **bold type** indicate severe, well-documented interactions.   †Canadian

INTERACTING AGENTS	POSSIBLE EFFECTS	NURSING CONSIDERATIONS
glyburide (continued)		
beta blockers, including ophthalmics	May mask symptoms of hypoglycemia.	• Monitor serum glucose level. • Monitor patient closely for signs of hypoglycemia, including dizziness, diaphoresis, confusion, and tachycardia. • Dosage adjustment may be needed.
hydantoins	May increase blood level of hydantoins.	• Monitor serum levels of these drugs.
alcohol	May alter glycemic control. May also cause disulfiram-like reactions of nausea, vomiting, abdominal cramps, and headaches.	• Advise patient to avoid alcohol.
smoking	May increase corticosteroid release; patient who smokes may require higher dosages of glipizide.	• Discourage smoking.
griseofulvin microsize • Fulvicin-U/F, Grifulvin V, Grisactin **griseofulvin ultramicrosize** • Fulvicin P/G, Grisactin Ultra, Gris-PEG		
barbiturates	May impair absorption of griseofulvin.	• Give these drugs at separate times. • Dosage may need to be increased.
cyclosporine salicylates	May decrease serum levels of these drugs.	• Monitor cyclosporine level, if appropriate. • Avoid salicylate combination, if possible. • Monitor for decreased therapeutic effects.
oral contraceptives	May decrease efficacy of contraceptives.	• Advise patient to use barrier contraception.

(warfarin)	*(...)*	- Dosage adjustment may be needed.
high-fat meals	May increase absorption.	- Drug may be given with a high-fat meal.
alcohol	May cause increase in alcohol effect, causing tachycardia, diaphoresis, and flushing.	- Advise patient to avoid alcohol.

guanabenz acetate • Wytensin

antihypertensives diuretics	May increase risk of excessive hypotension.	- Monitor BP frequently.
alcohol barbiturates benzodiazepines phenothiazines sedatives	May increase CNS-depressant effects.	- Should be used together cautiously. - Monitor patient closely for increased sedation, dizziness, ataxia, tremor, agitation, and respiratory depression. - Advise patient to avoid alcohol.
MAO inhibitors TCAs	May inhibit antihypertensive effects of guanabenz.	- Monitor BP frequently during initial therapy and when one drug is discontinued.

haloperidol • Apo-Haloperidol†, Haldol, Novo-Peridol†, Peridol†
haloperidol decanoate • Haldol Decanoate, Haldol Decanoate 100, Haldol LA†, haloperidol lactate, Haldol, Haldol Concentrate, Haloperidol Intensol

aluminum- and magnesium-containing antacids and antidiarrheals	May decrease drug absorption.	- Separate administration times by 2 hr.
antiarrhythmics disopyramide procainamide quinidine	May increase incidence of arrhythmias and conduction defects. Haloperidol serum level may be increased when given with quinidine.	- Use together cautiously. - Monitor vital signs and ECG closely. - When given with quinidine, haloperidol dosage may need to be reduced.

(continued)

INTERACTING AGENTS	POSSIBLE EFFECTS	NURSING CONSIDERATIONS
haloperidol (continued)		
atropine or other anticholinergics, including antidepressants, antihistamines, MAO inhibitors, meperidine, phenothiazines, and antiparkinsonians	May cause oversedation, paralytic ileus, visual changes, and severe constipation.	• Use these drugs together only when needed. • Monitor patient closely for adverse effects. • Dosage adjustment or withdrawal of drugs may be needed.
beta blockers	May inhibit haloperidol metabolism, increasing plasma level and toxicity.	• Avoid using together, if possible. • Dosage adjustment or withdrawal of drugs may be needed.
bromocriptine	Haloperidol antagonizes the therapeutic effect of bromocriptine on prolactin secretion.	• Monitor patient for clinical effect. • Bromocriptine dose may need to be increased.
centrally acting antihypertensives (such as clonidine, guanabenz, guanadrel, guanethidine, methyldopa, reserpine)	Inhibits BP response. When used with methyldopa, there may be adverse mental symptoms and increased sedation.	• Monitor BP carefully. • When used with methyldopa, monitor patient for psychological adverse effects. • Dosage adjustment or withdrawal of drugs may be needed.
CNS depressants, including analgesics, barbiturates, narcotics, tranquilizers, and general, spinal, or epidural anesthetics, or with parenteral magnesium sulfate	May increase CNS depression.	• Check for signs of increased CNS depression, including increased sedation, headache, dizziness, ataxia, confusion, agitation, and respiratory depression.
dopamine	May decrease vasoconstricting effects.	• Monitor patient's clinical response to dopamine.
levodopa	May decrease effectiveness and increase toxicity of levodopa.	• Monitor patient for clinical response to levodopa. Monitor patient for toxicity.
lithium	May cause severe neurologic toxicity with an encephalitis-like syndrome and a	• Monitor patient closely, especially during the first several weeks

	haloperidol.	
nitrates	May produce hypotension.	• Monitor BP frequently.
phenobarbital	May enhance renal excretion of haloperidol.	• Monitor patient for decreased therapeutic response to haloperidol. • Check for hyperpyrexia if haloperidol is used during barbiturate withdrawal.
phenytoin rifampin	May decrease haloperidol serum level.	• Monitor patient for clinical response. • Haloperidol decreases the seizure threshold; monitor patients with seizure history.
propylthiouracil	May increase risk of agranulocytosis.	• Monitor CBC.
sympathomimetics, including epinephrine, phenylephrine, and ephedrine (often found in nasal sprays), and appetite suppressants	May decrease stimulatory and pressor effects of these drugs.	• Monitor patient for clinical effect. • Epinephrine is not the drug of choice in emergent situations (such as severe hypotension) because haloperidol may block the vasopressor effects. Phenylephrine or norepinephrine may be used.
nutmeg	May cause loss of symptom control and interference with existing therapy for psychiatric illnesses.	• Advise patient to avoid using together.
smoking (heavy)	May increase metabolism of haloperidol.	• Discourage smoking.

heparin sodium • Heparin Lock Flush, Hep-Lock, Hep-Lock U/P, Liquaemin

cephalosporins oral anticoagulants penicillins platelet inhibitors **salicylates**	May increase anticoagulant effect.	• Monitor patient for increased bleeding or bruising tendencies. • Monitor INR, PT, and PTT.

(continued)

Interacting agents in **bold type** indicate severe, well-documented interactions. †Canadian

INTERACTING AGENTS	POSSIBLE EFFECTS	NURSING CONSIDERATIONS
heparin sodium (continued)		
antihistamines cardiac glycosides nicotine tetracyclines	May partially counteract the anticoagulant action of heparin.	• Monitor PTT. • Dosage adjustment may be needed.
garlic ginkgo motherwort red clover	May increase risk of bleeding.	• Advise patient against using together. • Advise patient to contact a health care professional before using an herbal preparation.
hydralazine hydrochloride • Apresoline, Novo-Hylazin		
diuretics antihypertensives	May increase hypotensive effects.	• Monitor BP.
diazoxide MAO inhibitors	May cause severe hypotension.	• Monitor BP frequently.
epinephrine	May decrease pressor response.	• Monitor patient closely for clinical response.
hydrochlorothiazide • Apo-Hydro†, Aquazide-H, Diuchlor H†, Esidrix, Hydro-chlor, Hydro-D, HydroDIURIL, Microzide, Mictrin, Neo-Codema†, Novo-Hydrazide†, Oretic, Urozide†		
amphetamine methenamine compounds (such as methenamine mandelate) quinidine	May increase alkaline urine, causing decreased urinary excretion of some amines. Urinary alkalization decreases the therapeutic efficacy of methenamine compounds.	• Monitor patient for toxic drug effects if given with amphetamine or quinidine. • Monitor urinary pH if given with methenamine compounds.
antihypertensives	May increase hypotensive effect.	• Monitor BP frequently. • Combination may be used therapeutically.

cholestyramine colestipol	May bind hydrochlorothiazide, preventing its absorption.	• Give drugs 1 hr apart.
diazoxide	May increase hyperglycemic, hypotensive, and hyperuricemic effects of diazoxide.	• Monitor patient closely for these effects.
lithium	May reduce renal clearance, elevating serum lithium level.	• Reduction in lithium dosage by 50% may be needed.
digoxin	Electrolyte disturbances may cause cardiac arrhythmias.	• Monitor serum potassium and magnesium levels.

hydroxychloroquine sulfate • Plaquenil

digoxin	May increase serum digoxin level.	• Monitor serum digoxin level. • Closely monitor patient for signs of digitalis toxicity, including fatigue, asthenia, dizziness, arrhythmias, visual disturbances, nausea, vomiting, and diarrhea.
kaolin magnesium trisilicate	May decrease absorption of hydroxychloroquine.	• Administer drugs at separate times.
prolonged, unprotected sun exposure	May cause drug-induced dermatoses.	• Advise patient to take precautions.

hydroxyurea • Droxia, Hydrea

didanosine indinavir stavudine	May cause fatal pancreatitis.	• Data from controlled clinical trials are still lacking. • Use with extreme caution and closely monitor patient.
fluorouracil	May cause neurotoxicity.	• Avoid using together, if possible. • If used together, monitor patient for headache, drowsiness, dizziness, mental confusion, and seizures.

Interacting agents in **bold type** indicate severe, well-documented interactions.   †Canadian

INTERACTING AGENTS	POSSIBLE EFFECTS	NURSING CONSIDERATIONS
hyoscyamine • Cystospaz **hyoscyamine sulfate** • A-Spas S/L, Anaspaz, Cystospaz-M, Levsin, Levsin Drops, Levsin/SL, Levsinex Timecaps		
amantadine antihistamines phenothiazines TCAs	May increase anticholinergic effects.	• Monitor for increased adverse effects, including headache, dizziness, confusion, irritability, tachycardia, mydriasis, dry mouth, constipation, urinary retention, and hot, dry skin. • Dosage adjustment may be needed.
antacids antidiarrheals	May decrease absorption of hyoscyamine.	• Hyoscyamine should be taken 1 hr before these agents.
haloperidol phenothiazines	May reduce antipsychotic effectiveness.	• Monitor patient for expected clinical effects. • Dosage adjustment may be needed.
ibuprofen • Advil, Children's Advil, Medipren, Motrin, Motrin IB, Nuprin, PediaProfen, Rufen, Trendar		
ACE inhibitors	May reduce response; may cause acute reduction in renal function.	• Monitor patient for clinical effect. • Monitor renal function studies.
antacids	May decrease absorption of ibuprofen.	• Patient should take drugs at separate times.
anticoagulants thrombolytics (coumarin derivatives, heparin, streptokinase, urokinase)	May increase anticoagulant effects.	• Monitor PT, PTT, and INR. • Monitor patient for increased bleeding tendencies. • Dosage adjustment may be needed.
anti-inflammatory drugs aspirin carbenicillin cefamandole	May increase risk of bleeding from inhibited platelet aggregation or adverse GI reactions, including ulceration and hemorrhage.	• Avoid using together, if possible. • Monitor patient very closely if ibuprofen is used with any of these drugs. • Monitor patient for increased GI com-

cefoperazone
corticosteroids
dextran
dipyridamole
mezlocillin
piperacillin
plicamycin
salicylates
sulfinpyrazone
ticarcillin
valproic acid

plaints, abdominal pain, melena, and increased bleeding or bruising tendencies.

aspirin	May decrease bioavailability of ibuprofen.	• Monitor patient for drug effect.
coumarin derivatives nifedipine phenytoin verapamil	Toxicity of these drugs may occur.	• Monitor PT, INR, and serum drug levels, if appropriate. • Monitor patient for signs of drug toxicity.
antihypertensives diuretics	May decrease effectiveness of these drugs; diuretics may increase nephrotoxicity.	• Monitor BP and renal function test results.
acetaminophen anti-inflammatory drugs gold compounds	May increase nephrotoxicity.	• Monitor renal function test results closely.
insulin oral antidiabetics	May potentiate hypoglycemic effects.	• Monitor serum glucose level closely. • Monitor patient for signs of hypoglycemia, including dizziness, diaphoresis, confusion, and tachycardia. • Dosage adjustment may be needed.

(continued)

INTERACTING AGENTS	POSSIBLE EFFECTS	NURSING CONSIDERATIONS
ibuprofen *(continued)*		
lithium methotrexate	May decrease renal clearance of these drugs.	• Check for signs of lithium toxicity: sedation, confusion, tremors, muscle stiffness, increased deep tendon reflexes, visual changes, nystagmus. • Check for signs of methotrexate toxicity: myelosuppression, anemia, nausea, vomiting, diarrhea, dermatitis, alopecia, melena, or fatigue. • Monitor serum levels of these drugs.
ibutilide fumarate • Corvert		
class IA antiarrhythmics (disopyramide, quinidine, procainamide) class III drugs (amiodarone, sotalol)	May increase the potential for prolonged refractoriness.	• Don't use together. Wait at least 5 half-lives of antiarrhythmics before giving ibutilide or 4 hr after last dose of ibutilide before giving antiarrhythmics.
digoxin	Supraventricular arrhythmias may mask the cardiotoxicity associated with an excessive digoxin level.	• Monitor serum digoxin level. • Monitor ECG.
antihistamines drugs that prolong QT interval H₁-receptor antagonists phenothiazines tetracyclic antidepressants TCAs	May increase the risk of proarrhythmia.	• Monitor ECG for prolonged QT interval and arrhythmias.
ifosfamide • Ifex		
chloral hydrate phenobarbital phenytoin	May increase the activity of ifosfamide by induction of hepatic microsomal enzymes, increasing the conversion of	• Be alert for possible combined drug actions, desirable or undesirable, even though ifosfamide has been used suc-

	ifosfamide to its active form.	cessfully with other drugs, including other cytotoxic drugs.

imipenem and cilastatin sodium • Primaxin I.M., Primaxin I.V.

chloramphenicol	May impede the bactericidal effects of imipenem.	• Give chloramphenicol a few hr after imipenem and cilastatin.
cyclosporine	May increase adverse CNS effects.	• Monitor patient for adverse CNS effects. • An alternative antibiotic may be considered.
ganciclovir	May cause generalized seizures to occur during combined imipenem and cilastatin and ganciclovir therapy.	• Avoid use together, if possible. • Monitor patient for seizure activity if used together.
probenecid	May prevent tubular secretion of cilastatin (but not imipenem) and prolong plasma cilastatin half-life.	• Avoid using together.

imipramine hydrochloride • Apo-Imipramine†, Impril†, Novopramine†, Tofranil
imipramine pamoate • Tofranil-PM

barbiturates	May induce imipramine metabolism and decrease therapeutic efficacy. May cause additive CNS depression.	• Monitor patient for clinical effects. • Monitor patient for increased sedation or respiratory depression. • Dosage adjustment may be needed.
beta blockers cimetidine methylphenidate oral contraceptives propoxyphene	May inhibit imipramine metabolism, increasing plasma level and toxicity.	• Monitor for imipramine toxicity, including excessive anticholinergic activity (agitation, confusion, hallucinations, hyperthermia, seizures, urinary retention, pupillary dilation, dry mucous membranes) followed by increased CNS-depressant effects (decreased or absent reflexes, sedation, respiratory depression, hypotension, arrhythmias, hypothermia).

(continued)

INTERACTING AGENTS	POSSIBLE EFFECTS	NURSING CONSIDERATIONS
imipramine hydrochloride *(continued)*		
centrally acting antihypertensives (such as **clonidine**, guanabenz, guanadrel, guanethidine, methyldopa, reserpine)	May decrease hypotensive effects of antihypertensives.	• Avoid using with clonidine. • When used with other drugs, monitor BP frequently, especially when therapy starts. • Alternative antihypertensives may be needed.
CNS depressants, including alcohol, analgesics, barbiturates, narcotics, tranquilizers, and anesthetics (oversedation); atropine or other anticholinergics, including antihistamines, meperidine, phenothiazines, and antiparkinsonians	May cause oversedation, paralytic ileus, visual changes, and severe constipation.	• Use these drugs together only when needed. • Monitor patient for increased sedation or respiratory depression. • Monitor patient for GI or visual complaints. • Dosage adjustment may be needed. • Advise patient to avoid alcohol.
disulfiram ethchlorvynol	May cause delirium and tachycardia.	• Observe patient closely for these adverse effects or other signs of psychoses.
haloperidol phenothiazines	May decrease metabolism of imipramine, causing an increased serum level.	• Monitor serum imipramine level and patient for signs of toxicity. • Dosage adjustment may be needed.
antiarrhythmics (quinidine, disopyramide, procainamide) pimozide thyroid hormones	May increase risk of arrhythmias and conduction defects.	• Monitor ECG closely when concurrent drug therapy begins.
sympathomimetics, including epinephrine, phenylephrine, and ephedrine (often found in nasal sprays)	May increase BP.	• Monitor BP frequently • Monitor patient for severe hypertension.

quinolones	May potentiate life-threatening cardiac arrhythmias.	• Don't use together.
MAO inhibitors	Hyperpyretic crises, seizures, and death may occur.	• Don't give imipramine with or within 2 wk of MAO inhibitor therapy.
warfarin	May prolong PT and cause bleeding.	• Monitor PT and INR. • Monitor patient for increased bleeding tendencies.
smoking (heavy)	May induce imipramine metabolism and decrease therapeutic efficacy.	• Discourage smoking.

indapamide • Lozol

amphetamines quinidine	Indapamide may turn urine slightly more alkaline and may decrease urinary excretion of some amines.	• Monitor patient for toxic drug effects.
antihypertensives	Indapamide may potentiate hypotensive effects.	• Monitor BP. • Combination may be used therapeutically.
cholestyramine colestipol	May bind indapamide, preventing its absorption.	• Give drugs 1 hr apart.
diazoxide	May increase hyperglycemic, hypotensive, and hyperuricemic effects of diazoxide.	• Avoid this combination, if possible. • Monitor patient closely for these effects. • If patient is diabetic, the insulin dose may need adjustment.
digoxin	May cause electrolyte disturbances and cardiac arrhythmias.	• Monitor serum potassium and magnesium levels. Monitor ECG.
lithium	May reduce renal clearance, elevating serum lithium level.	• Lithium dosage may need to be reduced by 50%.

(continued)

Interacting agents in **bold type** indicate severe, well-documented interactions.   †Canadian

INTERACTING AGENTS	POSSIBLE EFFECTS	NURSING CONSIDERATIONS
indapamide (continued)		
methenamine compounds (such as methenamine mandelate)	Urinary alkalization may decrease the therapeutic efficacy of methenamine compounds.	• Avoid using together. • Monitor urinary pH.
indinavir sulfate • Crixivan		
midazolam triazolam	Competition for CYP3A4 by indinavir may inhibit the metabolism of these drugs and create the potential for serious or life-threatening events, such as arrhythmias or prolonged sedation.	• Don't give these drugs with indinavir.
HMG-CoA reductase inhibitors (such as atorvastatin, cerivastatin, lovastatin, simvastatin)	May increase risk of myopathy, including rhabdomyolysis.	• Monitor patient for signs of myopathy and rhabdomyolysis (increased serum creatinine kinase level, muscle aches, weakness).
didanosine	A normal gastric pH may be needed for optimal absorption of indinavir.	• Give didanosine and indinavir at least 1 hr apart on an empty stomach.
itraconazole ketoconazole	May cause an increase in the plasma level of indinavir.	• Reduced dosage of indinavir is needed.
rifabutin	May increase plasma levels.	• Reduced dosage of rifabutin is needed.
rifampin	Rifampin is a potent inducer of CYP3A4, which could markedly diminish plasma level of indinavir.	• Use together isn't recommended.
ergot alkaloids	May increase risk of ergot toxicity (peripheral vasospasm, ischemia of the extremities).	• Don't use together.

| sildenafil | May cause severe hypotension. | • Use together cautiously.
• Sildenafil dosage should be reduced. |
| St. John's wort | May decrease blood level of indinavir by more than 50%. | • Warn patient against using together. |

indomethacin, indomethacin sodium trihydrate • Apo-Indomethacin†, Indameth, Indochron E-R, Indocid†, Indocin, Indocin SR, Novomethacin†

anticoagulants thrombolytics (coumarin derivatives, heparin, streptokinase, urokinase)	May increase anticoagulant effects.	• Monitor PT, PTT, and INR. • Monitor patient for increased bleeding tendencies. • Dosage adjustment may be needed.
alcohol anti-inflammatory drugs aspirin carbenicillin cefamandole cefoperazone corticosteroids dextran dipyridamole mezlocillin piperacillin plicamycin salicylates sulfinpyrazone ticarcillin valproic acid	May increase risk of bleeding from inhibited platelet aggregation or adverse GI reactions, including ulceration and hemorrhage.	• Don't use together, if possible. • Monitor patient very closely if used together. • Monitor patient for increased GI complaints, abdominal pain, and melena, and for increased bleeding or bruising tendencies. • Advise patient to avoid alcohol.
aspirin	May decrease bioavailability of indomethacin.	• Monitor patient for drug effect.

(continued)

INTERACTING AGENTS	POSSIBLE EFFECTS	NURSING CONSIDERATIONS
indomethacin, indomethacin sodium trihydrate *(continued)*		
coumarin derivatives nifedipine phenytoin verapamil	Toxicity of these drugs may occur.	• Monitor PT, INR, and serum drug levels, as appropriate. • Monitor patient for signs of drug toxicity.
antihypertensives diuretics	May decrease effectiveness of these drugs; diuretics may increase nephrotoxicity.	• Monitor BP and renal function studies.
acetaminophen anti-inflammatory drugs gold compounds	May increase nephrotoxicity.	• Monitor renal function studies closely.
insulin oral antidiabetics	May potentiate hypoglycemic effects.	• Monitor serum glucose level closely. • Monitor patient carefully for signs of hypoglycemia, including dizziness, diaphoresis, confusion, and tachycardia. • Dosage adjustment may be needed.
lithium methotrexate	May decrease renal clearance of these drugs.	• Check for signs of lithium toxicity: sedation, confusion, tremors, muscle stiffness, increased deep tendon reflexes, visual changes, or nystagmus. • Check for signs of methotrexate toxicity: myelosuppression, anemia, nausea, vomiting, diarrhea, dermatitis, alopecia, melena, or fatigue. • Monitor serum levels of these drugs.
senna	May block diarrheal effects.	• Advise patient not to use together. • Advise patient to contact health care professional before using herbs.

alcohol anabolic steroids **beta blockers** clofibrate fenfluramine MAO inhibitors salicylates tetracycline	May prolong hypoglycemic effect.	• Monitor serum glucose level closely. • Monitor patient carefully for signs of hypoglycemia, including dizziness, diaphoresis, confusion, and tachycardia. • Dosage adjustment may be needed.
corticosteroids dextrothyroxine sodium epinephrine thiazide diuretics	May diminish insulin response.	• Monitor serum glucose level. • Monitor patient for signs of hyperglycemia (fatigue, polyuria, polydipsia, weight loss, abdominal pain, altered mental status, tachycardia, hypotension, glucosuria, ketonuria). • Dosage adjustment may be needed.
basil bay bee pollen burdock ginseng glucomannan horehound marsh mallow myrrh sage	May affect glycemic control.	• Advise patient to avoid using together unless advised by health care provider. • Monitor serum glucose level. • Monitor patient for signs of hyperglycemia (fatigue, polyuria, polydipsia, weight loss, abdominal pain, altered mental status, tachycardia, hypotension, glucosuria, ketonuria) or hypoglycemia, including dizziness, diaphoresis, confusion, and tachycardia.
smoking	May decrease absorption of insulin administered S.C.	• Advise patient to avoid smoking within 30 minutes of insulin injection.
marijuana	May increase insulin requirements.	• Inform patient of this interaction.

INTERACTING AGENTS	POSSIBLE EFFECTS	NURSING CONSIDERATIONS
ipratropium bromide • Atrovent		
antimuscarinics, including ophthalmics	May produce additive effects.	• Use together cautiously and monitor patient for increased adverse effects.
fluorocarbon propellant–containing oral inhalants (such as adrenocorticoids, cromolyn, glucocorticoids, sympathomimetics)	Giving ipratropium and other fluorocarbon propellant–containing oral inhalants too close together may increase risk of fluorocarbon toxicity.	• A 5-min interval between administration is recommended. • Monitor patient closely.
jaborandi tree pill-bearing spurge	These herbs may decrease therapeutic effect of drug.	• Advise patient against using together. • Advise patient to contact a health care professional before using an herbal preparation.
irinotecan hydrochloride • Camptosar		
antineoplastics	May cause additive adverse effects, such as myelosuppression and diarrhea.	• Monitor hematologic studies. • Monitor patient's stool frequency. • Monitor serum electrolyte levels.
isoniazid (INH) • Isotamine†, Laniazid, Laniazid C.T., Nydrazid, PMS Isoniazid†		
antacids	May decrease oral absorption of INH.	• Administer antacid at least 1 hr before INH.
anticoagulants	May increase anticoagulant activity.	• Monitor PT and INR. • Dosage adjustment may be needed. • Monitor patient for increased bleeding tendencies.
benzodiazepines (such as diazepam) carbamazepine phenytoin	May cause INH-induced inhibition of metabolism and elevate serum levels, causing toxicity.	• Monitor serum drug levels as appropriate. • Monitor patient for increased adverse effects. • Dosage adjustment may be needed.

corticosteroids	May decrease INH efficacy.	• Monitor patient for clinical effects.
cycloserine	May increase hazard of CNS toxicity, drowsiness, and dizziness.	• Monitor patient for adverse neurologic effects; monitor patient for safety.
disulfiram	May cause coordination difficulties and psychotic episodes.	• Closely observe patient. • Disulfiram dose may need to be reduced or the drug stopped.
rifampin	May accelerate INH metabolism to hepatotoxic metabolites.	• Monitor liver function test results. • One or both drugs may need to be discontinued.
alcohol	May increase risk of INH-induced hepatitis and seizures.	• Advise patient to avoid alcohol.

itraconazole • Sporanox

benzodiazepines (midazolam, triazolam)	May increase plasma levels of these drugs, which may prolong hypnotic and sedative effects.	• Avoid using together. • CNS-depressive effects may persist for several days after discontinuing itraconazole.
calcium channel blockers	May cause edema.	• Monitor patient for adverse effects. • Dosage adjustment may be needed.
cyclosporine tacrolimus	Itraconazole may increase cyclosporine or tacrolimus plasma levels.	• Reduce dosages of these drugs by 50% when using itraconazole doses > 100 mg/day. • Monitor cyclosporine or tacrolimus levels. • Monitor renal function.
digoxin	May increase digoxin level.	• Monitor serum digoxin level before therapy starts and frequently thereafter.

(continued)

INTERACTING AGENTS	POSSIBLE EFFECTS	NURSING CONSIDERATIONS
itraconazole *(continued)*		
H$_2$ antagonists isoniazid phenytoin rifampin	May reduce plasma itraconazole level.	• H$_2$ antagonists should be given 2 hr after itraconazole. • Avoid using with isoniazid, rifampin, and phenytoin.
HMG-CoA reductase inhibitors	Itraconazole may inhibit hepatic metabolism of HMG-CoA reductase inhibitors, causing an increased plasma level of the HMG-CoA drug and a greater risk of adverse effects.	• Don't use together. • Rhabdomyolysis has been reported.
indinavir ritonavir	May cause altered plasma level of either drug.	• Use together cautiously. • Monitor patient for increased adverse effects of either drug.
oral hypoglycemic drugs	May cause severe hypoglycemia.	• Monitor patient carefully for signs of hypoglycemia, including dizziness, diaphoresis, confusion, and tachycardia. • Dosage adjustment may be needed.
phenytoin	May cause altered phenytoin metabolism.	• Monitor serum phenytoin level.
vinca alkaloids (vinblastine, vincristine)	May increase risk of vinca alkaloid toxicity.	• If possible, avoid concurrent use of these agents. • If unavoidable, monitor patient for signs of toxicity, including constipation, myalgia, or neutropenia.
warfarin	May enhance anticoagulant effect.	• Monitor PT and INR. Monitor patient for increased bruising or bleeding tendencies.
grapefruit juice	May decrease plasma level and therapeutic effect of itraconazole.	• Tell patient not to take drug with grapefruit juice.

ketamine hydrochloride • Ketalar

enflurane halothane	Halothane blocks the CV stimulatory effects of ketamine, causing myocardial depression, bradycardia, and hypotension.	• Use together very cautiously. • If used together, monitor vital signs and ECG closely. • Be prepared to correct bradycardia and hypotension.
barbiturates narcotics	May prolong recovery time.	• Monitor patient's vital signs, respiratory status, and ECG closely. • Dosage adjustment may be needed.
tubocurarine and nondepolarizing muscle relaxants	May increase neuromuscular effects; may prolong respiratory depression.	• Monitor patient for respiratory depression or distress. • Monitor dosing carefully. • Be prepared to provide life support.
thyroid hormones	May cause hypertension and tachycardia.	• Monitor patient for these effects. • Be prepared to treat these symptoms if patient becomes distressed.

ketoconazole • Nizoral

cyclosporine	Drug may raise serum levels as a result of interference with metabolism.	• Monitor cyclosporine and serum creatinine levels.
drugs that raise gastric pH (antacids, antimuscarinics, cimetidine, famotidine, ranitidine)	May decrease absorption of ketoconazole.	• Give these drugs 2 hr after ketoconazole.
hepatotoxic drugs	Drug may enhance toxicity.	• Monitor serum liver enzyme level. • Observe patient for signs of liver toxicity.

(continued)

Interacting agents in **bold type** indicate severe, well-documented interactions.   †Canadian

INTERACTING AGENTS	POSSIBLE EFFECTS	NURSING CONSIDERATIONS
ketoconazole (continued)		
oral sulfonylureas	Effects of sulfonylureas may be intensified.	• Monitor serum glucose level. • Monitor patient for signs of hypo-glycemia, including dizziness, diaphoresis, confusion, and tachycardia.
phenytoin	Serum levels of both drugs may be altered.	• Monitor patient's response to drug and monitor drug levels.
rifampin	May decrease serum level of ketoconazole to ineffective levels.	• Monitor patient for clinical effect of drug therapy.
tacrolimus	May increase plasma level of tacrolimus.	• Use with caution. • Monitor renal function and tacrolimus level.
alprazolam **triazolam**	May decrease metabolism of these drugs, leading to increased CNS depression and psychomotor impairment.	• Don't use together.
warfarin	May enhance anticoagulant effect.	• Monitor PT and INR frequently. • Monitor patient for increased bleeding tendencies.
alcohol	May cause a disulfiram-like reaction.	• Advise patient to avoid alcohol.
corticosteroids	May increase corticosteroid plasma level.	• Monitor patient for increased adverse effects associated with corticosteroid therapy.
yew preparations	May inhibit ketoconazole metabolism.	• Advise patient against using together. • Advise patient to contact a health care provider before using an herbal preparation.

vinca alkaloids (vinblastine, vincristine)	May increase risk of vinca alkaloid toxicity.	• If possible, avoid giving these drugs together. • If they must be used together, monitor patient for signs of toxicity, including constipation, myalgia, or neutropenia.

ketoprofen • Orudis, Orudis KT

drugs that inhibit platelet aggregation (such as aspirin, parenteral carbenicillin, cefamandole, cefoperazone, dextran, dipyridamole, mezlocillin, piperacillin, plicamycin, salicylates, sulfinpyrazone, ticarcillin, valproic acid, other anti-inflammatory drugs)	May cause bleeding problems.	• Avoid using together, if possible. • Monitor PT and INR. • Monitor patient very closely. • Monitor patient for increased bleeding or bruising tendencies. • Advise patient to avoid alcohol.
antihypertensives diuretics	May decrease effectiveness of these drugs; may increase nephrotoxic potential from diuretics.	• Monitor BP and renal function test results.
aspirin	May decrease the bioavailability of ketoprofen.	• Monitor patient for drug effect.
coumarin derivatives heparin nifedipine phenytoin streptokinase urokinase verapamil	May cause toxicity to occur; may increase risk of bleeding.	• Monitor PT and INR. • Monitor serum drug levels, if appropriate. • Monitor patient for signs of drug toxicity.
acetaminophen anti-inflammatory drugs gold compounds	May increase nephrotoxicity.	• Monitor renal function test results closely.

(continued)

INTERACTING AGENTS	POSSIBLE EFFECTS	NURSING CONSIDERATIONS
ketoprofen *(continued)*		
insulin oral antidiabetics	May potentiate hypoglycemic effects because of the influence of prostaglandins on glucose metabolism.	• Monitor serum glucose level closely. • Monitor patient carefully for signs of hypoglycemia, including dizziness, diaphoresis, confusion, and tachycardia. • Dosage adjustment may be needed.
lithium methotrexate	May decrease renal clearance of lithium and methotrexate.	• Check for signs of lithium toxicity: sedation, confusion, tremors, muscle stiffness, increased deep tendon reflexes, visual changes, and nystagmus. • Check for signs of methotrexate toxicity: myelosuppression, anemia, nausea, vomiting, diarrhea, dermatitis, alopecia, melena, and fatigue. • Monitor serum levels of these drugs.
alcohol anti-inflammatory drugs corticosteroids corticotropin salicylates	May cause GI ulceration and hemorrhage.	• Avoid using together, if possible. • Monitor patient very closely for increased GI complaints, abdominal pain, and melena. • Advise patient to avoid alcohol.
dong quai feverfew garlic ginger ginkgo horse chestnut red clover	May increase the risk of bleeding.	• Advise patient against using together. • Advise patient to contact a health care professional before using an herbal preparation.
St. John's wort dong quai	May increase risk of photosensitivity.	• Advise patient to avoid using these herbs during drug therapy.

| prolonged sun exposure | May increase the risk of photosensitive reaction. | • Advise patient to take precautions. |

ketorolac tromethamine • Toradol

diuretics	May decrease efficacy of diuretic; may increase risk of nephrotoxicity.	• Monitor renal function studies.
salicylates warfarin	May increase blood levels of salicylates or warfarin.	• Don't give salicylates with ketorolac. • Monitor PT and INR. • Monitor patient for increased bleeding tendencies.
NSAIDs	May elevate plasma level of ketorolac, with potential for cumulative adverse effects.	• Avoid using together.
lithium	May decrease renal clearance of lithium, increasing lithium level, with possible lithium toxicity.	• Avoid using together, if possible. • If given together, closely monitor lithium level. • Monitor patient for signs of toxicity, including sedation, confusion, tremors, muscle stiffness, increased deep tendon reflexes, visual changes, and nystagmus.
methotrexate	May elevate and prolong methotrexate level, possibly leading to toxicity.	• Avoid using together, if possible. • If using together, closely monitor methotrexate level. • Monitor patient for signs of toxicity, including myelosuppression, anemia, nausea, vomiting, diarrhea, dermatitis, alopecia, melena, and fatigue.

(continued)

INTERACTING AGENTS	POSSIBLE EFFECTS	NURSING CONSIDERATIONS
ketorolac tromethamine (continued)		
probenecid	May decrease clearance and increase level of ketorolac.	• Avoid using together.
alcohol	May increase GI effects, including ulceration and hemorrhage.	• Advise patient to avoid alcohol.
labetalol hydrochloride • Normodyne, Trandate		
beta-adrenergic agonists	Labetalol may antagonize bronchodilation produced by these drugs.	• Use together cautiously. • Increased beta-adrenergic dosages may be needed.
cimetidine	May increase bioavailability of oral labetalol.	• If used together, labetalol dosage may need adjustment.
antihypertensives diuretics	Labetalol may potentiate antihypertensive effects of these drugs.	• Closely monitor BP.
glutethimide	May decrease bioavailability of oral labetalol.	• Monitor BP response. • Labetalol dosage may need adjustment.
halothane	May cause synergistic antihypertension and significant myocardial depression.	• Monitor patient's BP closely. • Halothane level should not exceed 3%.
nitroglycerin	Labetalol blunts the reflex tachycardia produced by nitroglycerin without preventing its hypotensive effect. In patients with angina, additional antihypertensive effects may occur.	• Monitor BP closely.
TCAs	May increase incidence of labetalol-induced tremor. Also, may inhibit	• Monitor patient for increased adverse effects.

| | imipramine metabolism. | • Monitor patient taking imipramine for signs of imipramine toxicity. |

lactulose • Cephulac, Cholac, Chronulac, Constilac, Constulose, Duphalac, Enulose, Heptalac, Kristalose

| antibiotics
neomycin | May decrease lactulose effectiveness by eliminating bacteria needed to digest it into the active form. | • Monitor patient for clinical effect. |
| nonabsorbable antacids | May decrease lactulose effectiveness by preventing a decrease in the pH of the colon. | • Avoid using together. |

lamotrigine • Lamictal

carbamazepine phenobarbital phenytoin primidone	May decrease lamotrigine steady-state level.	• Monitor patient for clinical effects. • Dosage adjustment may be needed.
folate inhibitors (such as cotrimoxazole, methotrexate)	May be affected by lamotrigine because it inhibits dihydrofolate reductase, an enzyme involved in the synthesis of folic acid.	• Monitor patient closely because drug may have an additive effect.
valproic acid	May decrease lamotrigine clearance, which increases steady-state level of drug.	• Monitor patient closely for toxicity, including dizziness, headache, ataxia, somnolence, nausea, vomiting, diarrhea, and blurred vision.
sun exposure	May cause photosensitivity reactions.	• Advise patient to take precautions.

INTERACTING AGENTS	POSSIBLE EFFECTS	NURSING CONSIDERATIONS
lansoprazole • Prevacid		
ampicillin esters iron salts ketoconazole	Lansoprazole may interfere with the absorption of these drugs.	• Separate administration times.
sucralfate	May delay lansoprazole absorption.	• Give lansoprazole at least 30 min before sucralfate.
theophylline	May cause mild increase in theophylline excretion.	• Dosage adjustment may be needed.
male fern	May be inactivated in alkaline stomach environment.	• Advise patient against using together. • Advise patient to contact a health care professional before using an herb.
leflunomide • Arava		
activated charcoal cholestyramine	May decrease plasma level of leflunomide.	• These agents are sometimes used for this effect in treating overdose.
hepatotoxic drugs methotrexate	May increase risk of hepatotoxicity.	• Monitor liver enzyme levels, as appropriate. • Monitor patient for signs of hepatotoxicity (jaundice, fever, abdominal pain, clay-colored stools, tea-colored urine).
rifampin	May increase level of active leflunomide metabolite.	• Use together cautiously.
leucovorin calcium (citrovorum factor or folinic acid) • Wellcovorin		
fluorouracil	Leucovorin may increase toxicity of fluorouracil.	• May be used together for therapeutic purposes. • Monitor patient closely for increased toxicity.

phenobarbital phenytoin primidone	May decrease serum anticonvulsant level and increase frequency of seizures.	• Although this interaction has occurred solely in patients receiving folic acid, it should be considered when leucovorin is given. • Anticonvulsant dose may need to be adjusted.

levalbuterol hydrochloride • Xopenex

beta blockers	May cause reduced pulmonary effect of the drug and, possibly, severe bronchospasm.	• Don't use together, if possible. • If using together is necessary, a cardioselective beta blocker should be considered. • Administer with caution.
digoxin	May decrease digoxin level (up to 22%).	• Monitor serum digoxin level.
loop diuretics thiazide diuretics	May cause ECG changes and hypokalemia.	• Monitor serum electrolyte levels and ECG.
MAO inhibitors TCAs	May potentiate the action of levalbuterol on the vascular system.	• Give with extreme caution in patients being given MAO inhibitors or TCAs, or within 2 wk after discontinuing these drugs.
short-acting sympathomimetic aerosol bronchodilators epinephrine	May cause increased adverse adrenergic effects.	• To avoid serious CV effects, use additional adrenergics with caution. • Monitor vital signs and ECG for arrhythmias.

INTERACTING AGENTS	POSSIBLE EFFECTS	NURSING CONSIDERATIONS
levetiracetam • Keppra		
alcohol antihistamines benzodiazepines drugs that cause drowsiness narcotics TCAs	May cause severe sedation.	• Use together cautiously. • Monitor patient for increased sedation, dizziness, agitation, and asthenia. • Advise patient to avoid alcohol.
levodopa-carbidopa • Sinemet 10-100, Sinemet 25-100, Sinemet 25-250, Sinemet CR 25-100, Sinemet CR 50-200		
amantadine benztropine procyclidine trihexyphenidyl	Anticholinergics may reduce the tremor associated with Parkinson's disease, increasing therapeutic efficacy. However, these drugs may also exacerbate involuntary movements and delay levodopa absorption.	• Monitor patient for clinical effects. • Levodopa dosage may need to be increased or anticholinergic dose decreased.
anesthetics or hydrocarbon inhalation	May cause arrhythmias because of increased endogenous dopamine level.	• Stop levodopa 6 to 8 hr before giving anesthetics, such as halothane.
antacids containing calcium, magnesium, or sodium bicarbonate	May increase absorption of levodopa.	• Give antacids 1 hr after levodopa.
anticonvulsants (such as hydantoins, phenytoin) benzodiazepines haloperidol papaverine phenothiazines rauwolfia alkaloids thioxanthenes	May decrease therapeutic effects of levodopa.	• These drugs should be avoided. • If unavoidable, monitor for decreased effectiveness of levodopa-carbidopa.
antihypertensives	May increase hypotensive effect.	• Monitor BP.

bromocriptine	May produce additive effects.	• Reduced levodopa dosage may be needed.
MAO inhibitors	May cause a hypertensive crisis.	• Don't use together. • Discontinue MAO inhibitors for 2 to 4 wk before starting levodopa.
sympathomimetics	May increase risk of arrhythmias.	• Dosage reduction of the sympatho-mimetic is recommended. • Giving carbidopa with levodopa reduces the tendency of sympathomimetics to cause dopamine-induced arrhythmias. • Levodopa dose may need to be reduced.

levofloxacin • Levaquin, Quixin

antacids containing aluminum or magnesium iron salts zinc products sucralfate	May interfere with GI absorption of levofloxacin.	• Antacids may be safely given 2 hr before or 6 hr after levofloxacin. • Dietary supplements also shouldn't be given with levofloxacin.
antidiabetics	May alter blood glucose level.	• Monitor glucose level closely. • Monitor patient for signs of hypoglycemia. • Dosage adjustment may be needed.
NSAIDs	May increase CNS stimulation.	• Monitor patient for seizure activity.
warfarin and derivatives	May cause increased effect of oral anticoagulant with some fluoroquinolones.	• Monitor PT and INR. • Monitor patient for increased bleeding tendencies.

(continued)

Interacting agents in **bold type** indicate severe, well-documented interactions.   †Canadian

INTERACTING AGENTS	POSSIBLE EFFECTS	NURSING CONSIDERATIONS
levofloxacin *(continued)*		
theophylline	May decrease clearance of theophylline.	• Monitor theophylline level. • Monitor patient for increased adverse effects, including nausea, vomiting, dizziness, headache, agitation, confusion, seizures, tachycardia, arrhythmias, and respiratory failure.
sun exposure	May increase photosensitivity.	• Advise patient to take precautions.
levothyroxine sodium (T4 or L-thyroxine sodium) • Eltroxin, Levo-T, Levothroid, Levoxine, Levoxyl, Synthroid		
anticoagulants	May alter anticoagulant effect.	• Monitor PT and INR.
beta blockers (metoprolol, propranolol)	May increase pharmacologic effects.	• An increase in levothyroxine dosage may require a decrease in anticoagulant dosage.
cholestyramine	May delay absorption of levothyroxine.	• Hyperthyroidism increases the clearance of these drugs.
corticotropin	May cause changes in thyroid status.	• Dosage adjustment may be needed when patient achieves euthyroid state.
estrogens	May increase levothyroxine requirements.	• Don't administer together. • If used together, separate administration times by at least 6 hr.
hepatic enzyme inducers (such as phenytoin)	May increase hepatic degradation of levothyroxine and increase dosage requirements of levothyroxine.	• Monitor patient. • Dose adjustment of both drugs may be needed.
oral antidiabetics insulin	May alter serum glucose level. Administration of thyroid hormone may increase	• Monitor patient for decreased levothyroxine effect.

	insulin or antidiabetic requirements.	• Monitor patient for clinical effect. • Dosage adjustment may be needed.
somatrem	May accelerate epiphyseal maturation.	• Monitor serum glucose level when therapy starts and with any levothyroxine dosage change. • Dosage adjustment may be needed.
theophylline	May decrease theophylline clearance in hypothyroid patients.	• Don't use together in children, if possible.
TCAs sympathomimetics	May increase the effects of any or all of these drugs and may lead to coronary insufficiency or arrhythmias.	• Clearance returns to normal when euthyroid state is achieved. • Monitor patient closely for increased adverse effects (especially cardiac).

lidocaine (lignocaine) • Xylocaine
lidocaine hydrochloride • Anestacon, Dilocaine, L-Caine, Lidoderm Patch, Lidoject, LidoPen Auto-Injector, Nervocaine, Xylocaine, Xylocaine Viscous, Zilactin-L

beta blockers	May enhance sympathomimetic effects with lidocaine and epinephrine combination.	• Don't use together.
butyrophenones phenothiazines	May reduce or reverse the pressor effects of epinephrine.	• Avoid using together, if possible. If used together, monitor patient for drug effect.
beta blockers **cimetidine**	May cause lidocaine toxicity from reduced hepatic clearance.	• Monitor serum lidocaine level. • Monitor patient for signs of lidocaine toxicity, including somnolence, confusion, paresthesias, tinnitus, blurred vision, seizures, respiratory depression, hypotension, bradycardia, and arrhythmias.

(continued)

INTERACTING AGENTS	POSSIBLE EFFECTS	NURSING CONSIDERATIONS
lidocaine *(continued)*		
cyclic antidepressants MAO inhibitors	May cause prolonged and severe hypertension when lidocaine is used with epinephrine.	• Avoid using together.
succinylcholine	May increase neuromuscular effects of succinylcholine when used with high-dose lidocaine.	• Monitor patient for increased respiratory depression.
antiarrhythmics (including phenytoin, procainamide, propranolol, quinidine)	May cause additive or antagonist effects and additive toxicity.	• Monitor patient for clinical effects and for signs of toxicity.
ergot-type oxytoxic drugs vasopressor drugs	May cause severe, persistent hypertension or CVA when used with lidocaine and epinephrine combination.	• Avoid using lidocaine with epinephrine.
pareira	May add to or potentiate the effects of neuromuscular blockade.	• Avoid using together. • Advise patient to contact a health care professional before using an herb.
lisinopril • Prinivil, Zestril		
diuretics	May cause excessive hypotension.	• Monitor BP closely.
indomethacin	May attenuate the hypotensive effect of lisinopril.	• Monitor patient closely for BP response.
lithium	May increase serum lithium level.	• Monitor serum lithium level. • Monitor patient for signs of toxicity, including sedation, confusion, tremors, muscle stiffness, increased deep tendon reflexes, visual changes, and nystagmus.
potassium-containing salt substitutes potassium-sparing diuretics	May cause hyperkalemia.	• Monitor renal function and serum potassium level. Monitor patient for signs of

potassium supplements

nyperkalemia. Advise patient not to use
potassium salt substitutes.

lithium • Carbolith†, Duralith†, Eskalith, Lithane, Lithizine†, Lithobid, Lithonate, Lithotabs

antacids drugs containing aminophylline, caffeine, calcium, sodium, or theophylline	May increase lithium excretion by renal competition for elimination, decreasing therapeutic effect of lithium.	• Monitor patient closely for clinical re- sponse.
carbamazepine fluoxetine mazindol methyldopa phenytoin tetracyclines	May increase potential for lithium toxicity.	• Monitor serum lithium level. • Monitor patient for signs of toxicity, in- cluding sedation, confusion, tremors, muscle stiffness, increased deep tendon reflexes, visual changes, and nystagmus.
chlorpromazine phenothiazines	May decrease effects of chlorpromazine. Lithium and phenothiazines may cause disorientation, unconsciousness, and extrapyramidal symptoms.	• Monitor patient for clinical effects and increased adverse effects. • Interactions may be unpredictable.
electroconvulsive therapy (ECT)	Acute neurotoxicity with delirium has occurred in patients receiving lithium and ECT.	• Lithium dosage reduction or withdrawal of drug is needed before ECT.
haloperidol	May cause severe encephalopathy characterized by confusion, tremors, extrapyramidal effects, and weakness.	• Monitor patient very closely, especially during the first several wk.
indomethacin NSAIDs phenylbutazone piroxicam	May decrease renal excretion of lithium.	• Monitor serum lithium level. • May require a 30% reduction in lithium dosage.

(continued)

INTERACTING AGENTS	POSSIBLE EFFECTS	NURSING CONSIDERATIONS
lithium (continued)		
neuromuscular blockers (such as atracurium, pancuronium, succinylcholine)	May potentiate the effects of these drugs.	• Monitor patient closely for prolonged sedation or increased respiratory depression. • Dosage of these drugs may need to be reduced.
sympathomimetics, especially norepinephrine	Lithium may interfere with pressor effects of these drugs.	• Monitor patient closely for expected clinical response.
thiazide diuretics	May decrease renal excretion and enhance lithium toxicity.	• Monitor serum lithium level. • Diuretic dosage may need to be reduced by 30%.
dietary sodium	May alter renal elimination of lithium. Increased sodium intake may increase elimination of drug; decreased intake may decrease elimination.	• Monitor serum lithium level.
sibutramine parsley	May promote or produce serotonin syndrome (altered mental status; increased muscle tone, weakness, twitching; hyperthermia; delirium; coma; death).	• Concomitant use of these agents is not recommended. • Advise patient to contact a health care provider before using an herbal preparation.
psyllium seed	May inhibit GI absorption.	• Concomitant use of these agents is not recommended. • Advise patient to contact a health care provider before using an herbal preparation.
caffeine	May interfere with effectiveness of drug.	• Advise patient to avoid caffeine use.

lomefloxacin hydrochloride • Maxaquin

antacids minerals sucralfate	These drugs may bind with lomefloxacin in the GI tract and impair its absorption.	• Give antacids and sucralfate no less than 4 hr before or 2 hr after lomefloxacin.
cimetidine	Lomefloxacin may show substantially increased plasma half-lives.	• Monitor patient for signs of toxicity, including dizziness, headache, confusion, irritability, seizures, nausea, diarrhea, tinnitus, blurred vision, CV abnormalities, and dyspnea.
cyclosporine warfarin	Lomefloxacin may increase the effects or serum levels of these drugs.	• Monitor for toxicity. • Monitor serum levels, PT and INR, and renal function studies p.r.n.
probenecid	May decrease excretion of lomefloxacin.	• Don't give together, if possible. • If used together, consider this interaction.
sun exposure	May cause photosensitivity reactions.	• Advise patient to take precautions.

loperamide hydrochloride • Imodium, Imodium A-D, Kaopectate II, Maalox Anti-Diarrheal, Pepto Diarrhea Control

opioid analgesics	May cause severe constipation.	• Avoid using together. • If use can't be avoided, monitor patient for constipation, abdominal pain, and distention.

INTERACTING AGENTS	POSSIBLE EFFECTS	NURSING CONSIDERATIONS
lorazepam • Apo-Lorazepam†, Ativan, Novo-Lorazem†		
alcohol antidepressants antihistamines barbiturates general anesthetics MAO inhibitors narcotics phenothiazines	Lorazepam may potentiate the CNS-depressant effects of these drugs.	• Monitor patient closely for increased sedation, dizziness, ataxia, tremor, agitation, or respiratory depression. • Advise patient to avoid alcohol.
cimetidine disulfiram (possibly)	May diminish hepatic metabolism of lorazepam, which increases its plasma level.	• Monitor patient for increased adverse effects. • Lorazepam dosage may need to be reduced.
scopolamine	May be associated with an increased incidence of hallucinations, irrational behavior, and increased sedation.	• Monitor patient closely for these adverse effects.
smoking (heavy)	May accelerate lorazepam metabolism, lowering clinical effectiveness.	• Monitor patient for clinical effect. • Discourage smoking.
lovastatin • Mevacor		
cholestyramine colestipol	May enhance lipid-reducing effects but may decrease bioavailability of lovastatin.	• Separate administration times by at least 4 hr.
cyclosporine erythromycin gemfibrozil niacin	May increase risk of severe myopathy or rhabdomyolysis.	• Monitor patient for signs of myopathy and rhabdomyolysis (increased serum creatinine kinase level, muscle aches, weakness).

warfarin	May increase anticoagulant effect.	• Monitor PT and INR. • Monitor patient for increased bleeding tendencies.
isradipine	May increase clearance of lovastatin and its metabolites.	• Monitor patient for clinical effects. • Dosage adjustment may be needed.
itraconazole	May increase lovastatin level.	• Therapy with lovastatin should be temporarily interrupted if systemic azole antifungal treatment is required.
sun exposure	May cause photosensitivity reaction.	• Advise patient to take precautions.
alcohol	May increase hepatic effects.	• Advise patient to avoid alcohol.
grapefruit juice	May increase lovastatin serum level and increase adverse effects, such as rhabdomyolysis.	• Don't administer together.

magnesium hydroxide (milk of magnesia) • Milk of Magnesia, Phillips' Milk of Magnesia, Concentrated Phillips' Milk of Magnesia

chlordiazepoxide chlorpromazine dicumarol digoxin iron salts isoniazid	Using magnesium hydroxide with aluminum hydroxide may decrease the absorption rate of these drugs.	• Separate administration times.
enteric-coated tablets	May cause premature release of enterically coated drugs.	• Separate administration times.
quinolones tetracyclines	May decrease absorption.	• Separate administration times; for tetracyclines, give at least 3 to 4 hr apart; for quinolones, give the antacid ≥ 6 hr before or 2 hr after the quinolone dose.

INTERACTING AGENTS	POSSIBLE EFFECTS	NURSING CONSIDERATIONS
magnesium salicylate • Extra Strength Doan's, Magan, Mobidin		
ammonium chloride urine acidifiers	May increase magnesium salicylate serum level.	• Monitor patient for signs of magnesium salicylate toxicity, including metabolic acidosis with respiratory alkalosis, hyperpnea, tachypnea, tinnitus, nausea, and vomiting.
antacids urine alkalizers	May decrease magnesium salicylate serum level.	• Monitor patient for decreased salicylate effect.
anticoagulants thrombolytics	May potentiate platelet-inhibiting effects of magnesium salicylate.	• Dosage adjustment may be needed. • Monitor clinical effects as appropriate.
corticosteroids	May enhance magnesium salicylate elimination.	• Monitor patient for decreased salicylate effect.
drugs that are highly protein-bound (such as phenytoin, sulfonylureas, warfarin)	May cause displacement of either drug; possible adverse effects.	• Monitor patient for expected clinical effects and for signs of toxicity. • Monitor serum levels.
alcohol GI-irritant drugs (antibiotics, corticosteroids, NSAIDs)	May potentiate adverse GI effects of magnesium salicylate.	• Monitor patient for abdominal pain, GI distress, and melena. • Advise patient to avoid alcohol.
methotrexate	May increase toxic effects of methotrexate.	• Monitor patient for signs of toxicity, including myelosuppression, anemia, nausea, vomiting, diarrhea, dermatitis, alopecia, melena, and fatigue. • Monitor serum level.

mannitol • Osmitrol, Resectisol

cardiac glycosides	May enhance the possibility of digitalis toxicity.	• Monitor serum digoxin levels.
diuretics (including carbonic anhydrase inhibitors)	May increase effects of these drugs.	• Monitor patient closely. • Monitor serum electrolyte levels and patient's fluid balance.
lithium	May enhance renal excretion of lithium and lower serum lithium level.	• Monitor serum lithium levels.

mebendazole • Vermox

anticonvulsants (including carbamazepine and phenytoin)	May enhance the metabolism of mebendazole and decrease its efficacy.	• Monitor patient for clinical effect.
cimetidine	May inhibit mebendazole metabolism and may result in its increased plasma level.	• Monitor patient for increased GI disturbances and altered mental status.

megestrol acetate • Megace

bromocriptine	May cause amenorrhea or galactorrhea, interfering with the action of bromocriptine.	• Concurrent use isn't recommended.

meloxicam • Mobic

ACE inhibitors	May diminish antihypertensive effects.	• Monitor BP.
aspirin	May increase risk of adverse effects.	• Using together isn't recommended.
furosemide thiazide diuretics	NSAIDs may reduce sodium excretion associated with diuretics, leading to sodium retention.	• Monitor patient for edema and increased BP.

(continued)

INTERACTING AGENTS	POSSIBLE EFFECTS	NURSING CONSIDERATIONS
meloxicam *(continued)*		
lithium	May increase lithium level.	• Monitor serum lithium level closely.
warfarin	May increase PT or INR and increase risk of bleeding complications.	• Monitor PT and INR. • Monitor patient for increased bleeding tendencies.
alcohol smoking	May increase risk of GI irritation and bleeding.	• Monitor patient for increased abdominal pain, GI distress, and melena. • Advise patient against smoking and alcohol use.
meperidine hydrochloride (pethidine hydrochloride) • Demerol		
anticholinergics	May cause paralytic ileus.	• Monitor patient for abdominal pain, distension, decreased or absent bowel sounds, nausea, or vomiting.
cimetidine	May increase respiratory and CNS depression, causing confusion, disorientation, apnea, or seizures.	• Monitor patient's respiratory status. • Dosage reduction of meperidine or withdrawal of drug may be needed. • Be prepared to give a narcotic antagonist.
CNS depressants (such as narcotic analgesics, general anesthetics, antihistamines, barbiturates, benzodiazepines, muscle relaxants, phenothiazines, sedative-hypnotics, TCAs) alcohol	May potentiate respiratory and CNS depression, sedation, and hypotensive effects of drugs.	• Use together cautiously. • Monitor patient closely for increased sedation, dizziness, ataxia, tremor, agitation, respiratory depression, and hypotension. • Advise patient to avoid alcohol.
general anesthetics	May cause severe CV depression.	• Monitor vital signs and ECG closely.

isoniazid	Meperidine may potentiate adverse effects of isoniazid.	• Monitor patient for increased adverse effects.
MAO inhibitors	May precipitate unpredictable and occasionally fatal reactions, even in patients who may receive MAO inhibitors within 14 days of receiving meperidine.	• Avoid using together.
narcotic antagonist	Patient who becomes physically dependent on drug may experience acute withdrawal syndrome if given a narcotic antagonist.	• Avoid using together, if possible.
parsley	May promote or produce serotonin syndrome (altered mental status; increased muscle tone, weakness, twitching; hyperthermia; delirium; coma; death).	• Shouldn't be used together. • Advise patient against concomitant herbal use. • Advise patient to contact a health care professional before using an herb.
ritonavir	May cause significant increase in serum meperidine level.	• Avoid using together.

meropenem • Merrem I.V.

| propenecid | May compete with meropenem for active tubular secretion, inhibiting the renal excretion of meropenem. | • Avoid using together. |

metaproterenol sulfate • Alupent, Metaprel

| beta blockers | May antagonize bronchodilating effects of metaproterenol. | • Don't use together, if possible.
• If using together is necessary, a cardioselective beta blocker should be considered, but give with caution. |

(continued)

INTERACTING AGENTS	POSSIBLE EFFECTS	NURSING CONSIDERATIONS
metaproterenol sulfate *(continued)*		
cardiac glycosides general anesthetics (especially chloroform, cyclopropane, halothane, trichloroethylene) levodopa theophylline derivatives thyroid hormones	May increase the potential for cardiac effects, including severe ventricular tachycardia, arrhythmias, and coronary insufficiency.	• Use together cautiously. • Monitor vital signs and ECG for arrhythmias.
MAO inhibitors TCAs	May potentiate their CV actions.	• Give with extreme caution in patients being given MAO inhibitors or TCAs, or within 2 wk after discontinuing these drugs.
sympathomimetics	May cause additive effects and toxicity.	• To avoid serious CV effects and toxicity, avoid using additional sympathomimetics with metaproterenol. • Separate administration times. • Monitor vital signs and ECG for arrhythmias.
CNS stimulants sympathomimetics xanthines	May increase CNS stimulation.	• Monitor patient for signs of increased stimulation, including nervousness, anxiety, tremors, headache, and dizziness.
metformin hydrochloride • Glucophage		
calcium channel blockers corticosteroids diuretics estrogens isoniazid nicotinic acid	May cause hyperglycemia.	• Monitor serum glucose level. • Monitor patient for signs of hyperglycemia (fatigue, polyuria, polydipsia, weight loss, abdominal pain, altered mental status, tachycardia, hypotension, glucosuria, ketonuria).

oral contraceptives phenothiazines phenytoin sympathomimetics thiazides thyroid hormones		• Metformin dosage may need to be increased.
cationic drugs (such as amiloride, cimetidine, digoxin, morphine, procainamide, quinidine, quinine, ranitidine, triamterene, trimethoprim, vancomycin)	May compete for common renal tubular transport systems, which may increase metformin plasma level.	• Monitor serum glucose level closely. • Monitor patient carefully for signs of hypoglycemia, including dizziness, diaphoresis, confusion, and tachycardia. • Dosage adjustment may be needed.
nifedipine	May increase metformin plasma level.	• Monitor serum glucose level closely. • Monitor patient for signs of hypoglycemia. • Metformin dosage may need to be decreased.
iodinated contrast materials, parenteral	May increase risk of lactic acidosis.	• Don't give together. Metformin should be temporarily stopped 48 hr before procedure.

methadone hydrochloride • Dolophine, Methadose, Physeptone†

alcohol CNS depressants (such as narcotic analgesics, general anesthetics, antidepressants, antihistamines, barbiturates, benzodiazepines, muscle relaxants, phenothiazines, sedative-hypnotics)	May potentiate respiratory and CNS depression, sedation, and hypotensive effects.	• Use together cautiously. • Monitor patient closely for increased sedation, dizziness, ataxia, tremor, agitation, respiratory depression, and hypotension. • Advise patient to avoid alcohol.

(continued)

INTERACTING AGENTS	POSSIBLE EFFECTS	NURSING CONSIDERATIONS
methadone hydrochloride *(continued*		
cimetidine	May increase respiratory and CNS depression, causing confusion, disorientation, apnea, or seizures.	• Monitor patient's respiratory status. • Dosage reduction of methadone or withdrawal of drugs may be needed. • Be prepared to give a narcotic antagonist.
opioid antagonists	Patient who becomes physically dependent on drug may experience acute withdrawal syndrome if given with methadone.	• Avoid using together unless needed.
rifampin	May reduce blood level of methadone.	• Monitor patient for clinical effects. • Methadone dose may need to be increased.
methamphetamine hydrochloride • Desoxyn, Desoxyn Gradumets		
acetazolamide antacids sodium bicarbonate	May enhance reabsorption of methamphetamine and prolong duration of action.	• Monitor patient closely for increased adverse effects.
general anesthesia	May increase risk of arrhythmias.	• Avoid using together, if possible. • Monitor patient's vital signs and ECG closely.
antihypertensives	May antagonize their effects.	• Monitor BP.
ascorbic acid	May enhance methamphetamine excretion and shorten duration of action.	• Monitor patient for clinical effects. • Methamphetamine dose may need to be increased.
barbiturates	May antagonize methamphetamine by CNS depression.	• Monitor patient for clinical effects.

CNS stimulants	May cause additive effects.	• Avoid using together.
insulin	May alter insulin requirements in diabetic patient.	• Monitor serum glucose level. • Dosage adjustment may be needed.
MAO inhibitors (or drugs with MAO-inhibiting activity, such as furazolidone)	May cause hypertensive crisis.	• Avoid using together.
haloperidol phenothiazines	May decrease methamphetamine effects.	• Monitor patient for clinical effect.
SSRIs	May increase sensitivity to methamphetamine and increase risk of serotonin syndrome (altered mental status; increased muscle tone, weakness, twitching; hyperthermia; delirium; coma; death).	• Avoid use together, if possible. • If used together, monitor patient for increased CNS effects.
caffeine	May cause additive effects.	• Avoid using together.
melatonin	May enhance methamphetamine's monoaminergic effects and exacerbate insomnia.	• Advise patient against using together. • Advise patient to contact a health care professional before using an herb.

methimazole • Tapazole

anticoagulants	Antivitamin K action of methimazole may potentiate the action of anticoagulants.	• Monitor PT, PTT, and INR. • Monitor patient for increased bruising or bleeding tendencies.
bone marrow depressants	May increase risk of agranulocytosis.	• Monitor hematologic studies.
hepatotoxic drugs	May increase the risk of hepatotoxicity.	• Monitor liver function test results. • Monitor patient for signs of hepatotoxicity (jaundice, fever, abdominal pain, clay-colored stools, tea-colored urine).

(continued)

Interacting agents in **bold type** indicate severe, well-documented interactions.   †Canadian

INTERACTING AGENTS	POSSIBLE EFFECTS	NURSING CONSIDERATIONS
methimazole *(continued)*		
iodinated glycerol lithium potassium iodide	May potentiate hypothyroid and goitrogenic effects.	• Monitor patient for change in control of thyroid disease. • Dosage adjustment may be needed.
adrenocorticoids corticotropin	May require a dosage adjustment of the steroid when thyroid status changes.	• Monitor patient for change in control of thyroid disease. • Dosage adjustment may be needed.
beta blockers digoxin theophylline	May increase therapeutic effects of these drugs.	• Monitor serum levels as appropriate. • Dosage reductions may be needed as patient becomes euthyroid.
methotrexate, methotrexate sodium • Folex, Mexate, Mexate-AQ, Rheumatrex Dose Pack		
probenecid	May increase the therapeutic and toxic effects of methotrexate.	• Requires a lower dosage of methotrexate.
NSAIDs penicillins salicylates sulfonamides sulfonylureas	May increase the therapeutic and toxic effects of methotrexate by displacing methotrexate from plasma proteins, increasing the level of free methotrexate.	• Monitor methotrexate serum level. • Monitor patient for signs of methotrexate toxicity, including myelosuppression, anemia, nausea, vomiting, diarrhea, dermatitis, alopecia, melena, and fatigue. • Lower doses of methotrexate or prolonged leucovorin rescue may be needed.
immunizations	May not be effective when given during methotrexate therapy.	• Vaccines shouldn't be given during methotrexate therapy.
phenytoin	May increase risk of seizures.	• Monitor serum phenytoin level. • Phenytoin dosage may be increased.

folic acid	May decrease the effectiveness of methotrexate.	• Monitor patient for clinical effects.
pyrimethamine	Similar pharmacologic action.	• Don't use together.
oral antibiotics (such as chloramphenicol, tetracycline) nonabsorbable broad-spectrum antibiotics	May decrease absorption of methotrexate.	• Monitor serum methotrexate level. • Monitor patient for clinical effect.
potentially hepatotoxic drugs (such as retinoids, azathiopine, sulfasalazine)	May increase risk of hepatoxicity.	• Monitor liver function test results. • Monitor patient for signs of hepatotoxicity (jaundice, fever, abdominal pain, clay-colored stools, tea-colored urine).
sun exposure	May increase risk of photosensitivity reactions.	• Advise patient to use sunblock.

methyldopa • Aldomet, Apo-Methyldopa†, Dopamet†, Novomedopa†

anesthetics	May increase effects.	• Patient undergoing surgery may require reduced dosages of anesthetics.
antihypertensives	May potentiate antihypertensive effects.	• Monitor BP.
diuretics	May increase hypotensive effect of methyldopa.	• Monitor BP. • Dosage reduction may be needed.
haloperidol	May produce dementia and sedation.	• If these symptoms occur, one of the drugs needs to be discontinued.
ferrous gluconate ferrous sulfate	May decrease bioavailability of methyldopa, reducing hypotensive effects.	• Don't use these drugs together.
lithium	May increase risk of lithium toxicity.	• Monitor serum lithium level. • Monitor patient for signs of toxicity, including sedation, confusion, tremors,

(continued)

INTERACTING AGENTS	POSSIBLE EFFECTS	NURSING CONSIDERATIONS
methyldopa (continued)		
		muscle stiffness, increased deep tendon reflexes, visual changes, nystagmus.
phenothiazines TCAs	May reduce antihypertensive effects.	• Monitor BP.
phenoxybenzamine	May cause reversible urinary incontinence.	• Avoid using together.
sympathomimetics	May potentiate pressor effects.	• Monitor BP. • Sympathomimetic may be discontinued if significant hypertension develops.
tolbutamide	Methyldopa may impair tolbutamide metabolism.	• Monitor serum glucose level.
capsicum	May reduce antihypertensive effectiveness of drug.	• Advise patient against using together. • Advise patient to contact a health care professional before using an herbal preparation.
methylphenidate hydrochloride • Ritalin, Ritalin-SR, Concerta, Methylin, Metadate		
anticonvulsants (phenobarbital, phenytoin, primidone) coumarin anticoagulants phenylbutazone TCAs	Methylphenidate may inhibit metabolism and increase the serum levels of these drugs.	• Dosage adjustment may be needed.
bretylium guanethidine	May decrease hypotensive effects.	• Monitor BP and cardiac rhythm.
MAO inhibitors (or drugs with MAO-inhibiting activity) or within 14 days of such therapy	May cause severe hypertension.	• Monitor BP closely.

caffeine	May enhance CNS-stimulant effects of methylphenidate and decrease effectiveness of drug in attention-deficit hyperactivity disorder.	• Advise patient or parent to avoid use together.

methylprednisolone • Medrol

amphotericin B diuretic therapy	May enhance hypokalemia.	• Monitor serum potassium level. • Monitor patient for signs of hypokalemia, including muscle weakness, fatigue, nausea, vomiting, constipation, respiratory depression, and arrhythmias.
antacids cholestyramine colestipol	May decrease corticosteroid effect.	• Separate administration times.
anticholinesterase	May antagonize effects of anticholinesterases used in myasthenia gravis with resulting profound muscle weakness.	• Corticosteroids may have therapeutic benefits in these patients. • Monitor patient closely and have life support readily available.
oral anticoagulants	May decrease effectiveness.	• Monitor PT and INR.
barbiturates phenytoin **rifampin**	May cause decreased corticosteroid effects because of increased hepatic metabolism.	• Don't use together, if possible. • If unavoidable, monitor patient for loss of therapeutic effects. • The corticosteroid dosage may need to be increased.
cyclosporine	May increase level of cyclosporine.	• Monitor cyclosporine level.
estrogens	May reduce metabolism of corticosteroids.	• Dosage adjustment may be needed.

(continued)

INTERACTING AGENTS	POSSIBLE EFFECTS	NURSING CONSIDERATIONS
methylprednisolone *(continued)*		
insulin oral antidiabetics	Hyperglycemia may occur.	• Monitor serum glucose level. • Monitor patient for signs of hyperglycemia (fatigue, polyuria, polydipsia, weight loss, abdominal pain, altered mental status, tachycardia, hypotension, glucosuria, ketonuria).
isoniazid salicylates	May increase metabolism of these drugs.	• Dosage adjustment of isoniazid or salicylates may be needed.
ulcerogenic drugs such as NSAIDs	May increase risk of GI ulceration.	• Monitor patient for increased GI complaints, abdominal pain, or melena. • Use together cautiously.
vaccines	May decrease effectiveness of vaccines.	• Vaccines shouldn't be given during steroid therapy.
metoclopramide hydrochloride • Apo-Metoclop†, Clopra, Maxeran†, Maxolon, Octamide PFS, Reclomide, Reglan		
anticholinergics opiates	May antagonize effect of metoclopramide on GI motility.	• Avoid using together, if possible. • If used together, monitor patient for clinical effects.
alcohol CNS depressants (such as sedatives and TCAs)	May lead to increased CNS depression.	• Monitor patient closely for increased sedation, dizziness, ataxia, tremor, agitation, or respiratory depression. • Advise patient to avoid alcohol.
butyrophenone antipsychotics phenothiazine	May potentiate extrapyramidal reactions.	• Avoid using together, if possible.
cyclosporine	May increase absorption, possibly increasing its immunosuppressive and toxic effects.	• Monitor cyclosporine serum level. • Monitor patient for increased adverse effects.

digoxin	May decrease absorption.	• Monitor serum digoxin level.
MAO inhibitors	May increase BP.	• Avoid using together.

metolazone • Mykrox, Zaroxolyn

amphetamines quinidine	May decrease urinary excretion.	• Monitor patient closely for toxic drug effects.
antihypertensives	May potentiate effects.	• Combination may be used to therapeutic advantage.
cholestyramine colestipol	May bind metolazone, preventing its absorption.	• Give drugs 1 hr apart.
diazoxide	Metolazone may potentiate hyperglycemic, hypotensive, and hyperuricemic effects of diazoxide.	• Avoid this combination, if possible. • Monitor patient closely for these effects; if patient is diabetic, the insulin dose may need adjustment.
digoxin	May increase risk of digoxin toxicity.	• Monitor serum electrolyte levels and serum digoxin level. • Monitor ECG for arrhythmias.
furosemide	May cause excessive volume and electrolyte depletion.	• Monitor fluid and electrolytes.
insulin sulfonylurea	May increase requirements in diabetic patients.	• Monitor serum glucose level. • Monitor patient for signs of hyperglycemia (fatigue, polyuria, polydipsia, weight loss, abdominal pain, altered mental status, tachycardia, hypotension, glucosuria, ketonuria). • Dosage adjustment may be needed.

(continued)

INTERACTING AGENTS	POSSIBLE EFFECTS	NURSING CONSIDERATIONS
metolazone *continued*		
lithium	May elevate serum lithium level.	• A 50% reduction in lithium dosage may be needed.
methenamine mandelate	Urinary alkalization decreases the therapeutic efficacy of methenamine compounds.	• Avoid using together. • Monitor urinary pH if necessary to give with methenamine compounds.
sun exposure	May increase risk of photosensitivity reactions.	• Advise patient to use adequate protection or avoid excessive sun exposure.
metoprolol succinate • Toprol XL **metoprolol tartrate** • Lopressor		
cardiac glycosides	May enhance bradycardia.	• Monitor patient's apical pulse.
antihypertensives diuretics	May potentiate antihypertensive effects.	• This effect may be used for a therapeutic advantage. • Monitor BP closely.
sympathomimetics	Antagonizes beta-adrenergic effects of sympathomimetics.	• Monitor patient for clinical effect.
verapamil	Has additive effects. May cause a significant increase in metoprolol bioavailability.	• Don't use together, if possible. • If used together, monitor cardiac function. • Dosage adjustments may be needed.
clonidine	May cause life-threatening hypertension.	• Monitor patient's BP closely when these drugs are used together and after one is stopped.

metronidazole • Apo-Metronidazole†, Flagyl, Flagyl ER, Metric-21, Novonidazol†, Protostat
metronidazole hydrochloride • Flagyl I.V., Flagyl I.V. RTU, Metro I.V.

oral anticoagulants	May prolong PT and INR.	• Monitor patient for this effect. • Monitor patient for increased bleeding tendencies.
barbiturates phenytoin	May reduce antimicrobial effectiveness of metronidazole.	• May require higher doses of metronidazole.
cimetidine	May decrease clearance of metronidazole.	• Monitor patient for adverse effects.
disulfiram	May precipitate psychosis and confusion.	• Don't use together.
lithium	May increase lithium level.	• Monitor serum lithium level. • Monitor patient for signs of toxicity, including sedation, confusion, tremors, muscle stiffness, increased deep tendon reflexes, visual changes, and nystagmus.
alcohol	May cause disulfiram-like reaction (nausea, vomiting, headache, abdominal cramps, and flushing).	• Advise patient of this interaction. • Advise patient to avoid alcohol.

mexiletine hydrochloride • Mexitil

ammonium chloride	May enhance mexiletine excretion from increased urinary pH.	• Monitor patient for expected clinical effects. • Monitor plasma levels. • Dosage adjustment may be needed.
antacids containing aluminum-magnesium hydroxide atropine narcotics	May delay mexiletine absorption.	• Separate administration times.

(continued)

INTERACTING AGENTS	POSSIBLE EFFECTS	NURSING CONSIDERATIONS
mexiletine *(continued)*		
carbonic anhydrase inhibitors high-dose antacids sodium bicarbonate	May decrease mexiletine excretion.	• Monitor patient for signs of toxicity, including nausea, hypotension, cardiac arrhythmias, dizziness, headache, confusion, paresthesias, and seizures.
cimetidine	May increase or decrease mexiletine metabolism, causing altered serum levels.	• Monitor patient for clinical effects and signs of toxicity.
metoclopramide	May increase absorption.	• Separate administration times. • Monitor patient for increased adverse effects.
phenobarbital phenytoin rifampin	May induce hepatic metabolism of mexiletine and reduce serum drug levels.	• Monitor mexiletine serum level. • Monitor patient for clinical effects.
theophylline	May increase serum theophylline level.	• Monitor serum theophylline level. • Monitor patient for signs of toxicity, including nausea, vomiting, insomnia, irritability, tachycardia, arrhythmias, tachypnea, and seizures.
caffeine	May decrease caffeine metabolism.	• Advise patient to avoid caffeine use.
mezlocillin sodium • Mezlin		
aminoglycoside antibiotics	May cause synergistic bactericidal effect against *Pseudomonas aeruginosa, Escherichia coli, Klebsiella, Citrobacter, Enterobacter, Serratia,* and *Proteus mirabilis.*	• This is a therapeutic advantage. May be used for this effect.

clavulanic acid	May cause synergistic bactericidal effect against certain beta-lactamase–producing bacteria.	• This is a therapeutic advantage.
methotrexate	May delay elimination and elevate serum level of methotrexate.	• Monitor patient for methotrexate toxicity. • Monitor serum level. • An alternative antibiotic may be needed.
probenecid	May block tubular secretion of penicillins, raising their serum levels.	• Probenecid may be used for this purpose.
tetracyclines	May reduce penicillin effectiveness.	• Avoid using together.
vecuronium bromide	May prolong neuromuscular blockade.	• Monitor vital signs, ECG, and respiratory status.

midazolam hydrochloride • Versed

alcohol antidepressants antihistamines barbiturates CNS and respiratory depressants narcotics tranquilizers	May potentiate effects.	• Monitor patient closely for increased sedation, headache, dizziness, ataxia, confusion, agitation, respiratory depression, or other signs of CNS depression. • Midazolam dosage may be decreased. • Advise patient to avoid alcohol.
diltiazem erythromycin fluconazole HIV protease inhibitors itraconazole ketoconazole verapamil	May decrease plasma clearance of midazolam from inhibition of CYP3A4 isoenzyme.	• Monitor patient for prolonged sedation and respiratory depression; dosage adjustment may be needed. • Avoid use of midazolam with protease inhibitors.

(continued)

INTERACTING AGENTS	POSSIBLE EFFECTS	NURSING CONSIDERATIONS
midazolam hydrochloride *(continued)*		
droperidol fentanyl narcotics	May potentiate the hypnotic effect of mida- zolam.	• Monitor patient closely for increased se- dation. • Dosage adjustment may be needed.
inhaled anesthetics	Midazolam may decrease the needed dose of inhaled anesthetics by depressing respiratory drive.	• Anesthesia dosage may require adjust- ment.
isoniazid	May decrease the metabolism of midazo- lam.	• Monitor patient for increased adverse ef- fects.
carbamazepine phenobarbital phenytoin rifampin	May decrease plasma level of midazolam.	• Monitor for clinical effect. • Dosage adjustment may be needed.
grapefruit juice	May increase bioavailability of oral syrup form of drug.	• Give with other liquids.
minocycline hydrochloride • Dynacin, Minocin, Vectrin		
antacids containing aluminum, calcium, or magnesium dairy products foods laxatives containing magnesium milk **oral iron products** sodium bicarbonate	May decrease oral absorption of minocy- cline because of chelation.	• Separate administration times by 3 to 4 hr. • Enteric-coated or sustained-release iron preparations may be given with minocy- cline. • Antibiotic should be given 1 hr before or 2 hr after food and dairy products.
oral anticoagulants	May enhance anticoagulation effects.	• Monitor PT and INR. • Dose adjustment may be needed.

		• Monitor patient for increased bleeding tendencies.
oral contraceptives	May be less effective when given with minocycline.	• Advise patient to use barrier contraception.
cimetidine	May decrease absorption of minocycline.	• Monitor patient's clinical response. • Dose adjustment of minocycline may be needed.
digoxin	May increase bioavailability of digoxin	• Monitor serum digoxin level. • Monitor patient for signs of digoxin toxicity, including fatigue, asthenia, dizziness, arrhythmias, visual disturbances, nausea, vomiting, and diarrhea. • Dosage adjustment may be needed.
methoxyflurane	May increase risk of nephrotoxicity.	• Avoid using together.
penicillins	Tetracyclines may antagonize bactericidal effects of penicillin.	• Avoid giving these drugs together. • If unavoidable, administer penicillin 2 to 3 hr before tetracycline. • Monitor patient for expected clinical effects.
sun exposure	May increase risk of photosensitivity reactions.	• Advise patient to use sunblock and limit sun exposure.

minoxidil (systemic) • Loniten

diuretics hypotensives	May increase hypotensive effects.	• Combination may be used to therapeutic advantage.
guanethidine	May cause profound orthostatic hypotension.	• Discontinue guanethidine 1 to 3 days before starting minoxidil.

(continued)

INTERACTING AGENTS	POSSIBLE EFFECTS	NURSING CONSIDERATIONS
modafinil • Provigil		
inducers of CYP3A4 (carbamazepine, phenobarbital, rifampin) inhibitors of CYP3A4 (itraconazole, ketoconazole)	May alter level of modafinil.	• Monitor patient for increased adverse reactions and toxicity (anxiety, nervousness, insomnia, tremor, irritability, confusion, palpitations, nausea, diarrhea). • Dosage adjustment may be needed.
cyclosporine theophylline	May reduce serum levels of these drugs.	• Monitor serum drug levels. • Monitor patient for expected clinical effects.
diazepam, phenytoin, propranolol, or other agents metabolized by CYP2C19	May increase serum levels of drugs metabolized by this enzyme.	• Use together cautiously. • Dosage adjustment may be needed.
methylphenidate	May delay absorption of modafinil by about 1 hr.	• Separate dosage administration times.
phenytoin warfarin	May increase serum levels of these drugs.	• Monitor serum phenytoin level, PT, and INR as appropriate. • Monitor patient closely for signs of toxicity.
steroidal contraceptives	May reduce contraceptive effectiveness.	• Recommend alternative or concomitant method of contraception during modafinil therapy and for 1 mo after drug is stopped.
TCAs (such as clomipramine and desipramine)	Modafinil may increase levels.	• Dosage reduction of these drugs may be needed.

moexipril hydrochloride • Univasc

diuretics	May increase risk of excessive hypotension.	• Diuretic or lower dose of moexipril may be needed.
lithium	May cause lithium toxicity.	• Monitor lithium level. • Check for signs of toxicity, including sedation, confusion, tremors, muscle stiffness, increased deep tendon reflexes, visual changes, and nystagmus.
licorice	May cause sodium retention and increase BP, interfering with the therapeutic effects of ACE inhibitors.	• Discourage use together.
potassium-sparing diuretics potassium supplements sodium substitutes containing potassium	May increase risk of hyperkalemia.	• Monitor renal function test results and serum potassium level. • Monitor patient for signs of hyperkalemia. Caution patient to avoid salt substitutes.

molindone hydrochloride • Moban

alcohol	May have additive effects.	• Advise patient to avoid alcohol.
sun exposure	May increase risk of photosensitivity reactions.	• Advise patient to use sunblock and avoid excessive exposure to the sun.

moricizine hydrochloride • Ethmozine

cimetidine	May decrease moricizine clearance by 49%; no significant changes in efficacy or tolerance have been observed.	• Patient should receive decreased doses of cimetidine ($\leq$ 600 mg/day).
digoxin	May prolong the PR interval.	• Monitor ECG.

(continued)

Interacting agents in **bold type** indicate severe, well-documented interactions. †Canadian

INTERACTING AGENTS	POSSIBLE EFFECTS	NURSING CONSIDERATIONS
moricizine hydrochloride *(continued)*		
diltiazem	May increase moricizine level and decrease diltiazem level.	• Monitor patient for clinical effects. • Dosage adjustments may be needed.
propranolol	May produce a small additive increase in the PR interval.	• Monitor ECG.
theophylline	May increase theophylline clearance and decrease plasma half-life.	• Monitor serum theophylline level.
morphine hydrochloride† • Morphitec†, M.O.S.† **morphine sulfate** • Astramorph PF, Duramorph, Epimorph†, Infumorph, Kadian, MS Contin, MSIR, MS/L, MS/S, OMS Concentrate, Oramorph SR, RMS Uniserts, Roxanol, Statex†		
general anesthetics	May cause severe CV depression.	• Monitor vital signs and ECG closely.
anticholinergics	May cause paralytic ileus.	• Monitor patient for abdominal pain, distension, decreased or absent bowel sounds, nausea, or vomiting.
cimetidine	May increase respiratory and CNS depression.	• Dosage of morphine may need to be reduced or one or both drugs stopped. • Be prepared to give a narcotic antagonist.
alcohol CNS depressants (such as narcotic analgesics, general anesthetics, antihistamines, barbiturates, benzodiazepines, MAO inhibitors, muscle relaxants, phenothiazines, sedative-hypnotics, TCAs)	May potentiate respiratory and CNS depression, sedation, and hypotensive effects of drug.	• Use together cautiously. • Monitor patient closely for increased sedation, dizziness, ataxia, tremor, agitation, respiratory depression, and hypotension. • Advise patient to avoid alcohol.

narcotic antagonists	Patient who becomes physically dependent on this drug may experience acute withdrawal syndrome if given a narcotic antagonist.	• Avoid using together unless needed.
rifamycins	May decrease analgesic effect.	• Monitor patient for expected clinical effect. • Alternative analgesic may be needed.

moxifloxacin hydrochloride • Avelox

antacids didanosine metal cations (such as aluminum, magnesium, iron, zinc) multivitamins sucralfate	May cause interference with GI absorption of moxifloxacin; metal cations chelate with moxifloxacin, resulting in decreased absorption and lower serum levels.	• Give drug at least 4 hr before or 8 hr after any of these agents.
antipsychotics erythromycin TCAs	May have additive effect.	• Monitor patient and ECG closely. • Use with caution.
class IA (such as procainamide, quinidine) or Class III (such as amiodarone, sotalol) antiarrhythmics	Lack of clinical experience. These drugs may have the potential to prolong the QT interval when taken with moxifloxacin.	• Avoid using together.
NSAIDs	May increase risk of CNS stimulation and seizures.	• Avoid using together, if possible. • If used together, monitor patient for seizure activity.
sun exposure	Although photosensitivity hasn't occurred with moxifloxacin, it has been reported with other fluoroquinolones.	• Advise patient to use sunblock.

Interacting agents in **bold type** indicate severe, well-documented interactions.   †Canadian

INTERACTING AGENTS	POSSIBLE EFFECTS	NURSING CONSIDERATIONS
nadolol • Corgard		
antiarrhythmics	May have additive or antagonistic cardiac effects and additive toxic effects.	• Monitor patient for clinical effect and for potential increased adverse effects.
antihypertensives neuromuscular blockers (such as tubocurarine) diuretics	May potentiate antihypertensive effects. High doses of nadolol may prolong effects of neuromuscular blockers.	• This effect may be used for a therapeutic advantage. • Monitor BP closely. • When used with neuromuscular blockers, monitor patient for prolonged effects.
sympathomimetics (such as isoproterenol and **epinephrine)**	May antagonize beta-adrenergic effects of sympathomimetics. Using with epinephrine may cause 1st- or 2nd-degree heart block and hypertension.	• Monitor patient for clinical effect. • Monitor ECG and BP closely.
verapamil	May have additive effects.	• Monitor cardiac function. • Dosage adjustments may be needed.
clonidine	May cause potentially life-threatening hypertension.	• Monitor patient's BP closely when these drugs are used together and after one is stopped.
cocaine	May inhibit therapeutic effects of nadolol.	• Advise patient of this interaction.
nafcillin sodium • Nafcil, Nallpen, Unipen		
aminoglycosides	May produce synergistic bactericidal effects against *S. aureus*. However, the drugs are physically and chemically incompatible and are inactivated when mixed or given together.	• Don't mix in same solution.

cyclosporines	May cause subtherapeutic cyclosporine level.	• Monitor cyclosporine level.
hepatotoxic drugs	May increase the risk of hepatotoxicity.	• Monitor liver enzyme level as needed. • Monitor patient for signs of hepatotoxicity (jaundice, fever, abdominal pain, clay-colored stools, tea-colored urine).
tetracyclines	May reduce penicillin effectiveness.	• Avoid using together.
carbonated beverages fruit juice	Acidity may inactivate drug.	• Give with other liquids.

nalbuphine hydrochloride • Nubain

general anesthetics	May cause severe CV depression.	• Monitor vital signs and ECG closely.
barbiturate anesthetics (such as thiopental)	May cause additive CNS and respiratory depressant effects and, possibly, apnea.	• Monitor vital signs and respiratory status very carefully. • Barbiturate anesthetic dose may be lower.
cimetidine	May increase narcotic nalbuphine toxicity.	• A narcotic antagonist may be needed if toxicity occurs.
CNS depressants (antihistamines, barbiturates, benzodiazepines, muscle relaxants, narcotic analgesics, phenothiazines, sedative-hypnotics, TCAs)	May potentiate respiratory and CNS depression, sedation, and hypotensive effects.	• Use together cautiously. • Monitor patient closely for increased sedation, dizziness, ataxia, tremor, agitation, respiratory depression, and hypotension. • Reduced doses of nalbuphine are usually needed.
digitoxin phenytoin rifampin	May cause drug accumulation and enhanced effects.	• Monitor serum digoxin or phenobarbital level. • Monitor patient for signs of toxicity.

(continued)

Interacting agents in **bold type** indicate severe, well-documented interactions.   †Canadian

INTERACTING AGENTS	POSSIBLE EFFECTS	NURSING CONSIDERATIONS
nalbuphine hydrochloride (continued)		
narcotic antagonists	Patient who becomes physically dependent on drug may experience acute withdrawal syndrome if given high doses of a narcotic antagonist.	• Avoid using together unless needed.
naloxone hydrochloride • Narcan		
cardiotoxic drugs	May have serious CV effects.	• Use together cautiously. • Monitor patient for changes in BP, arrhythmias, and pulmonary edema.
nandrolone decanoate • Androlone-D 200, Deca-Durabolin, Hybolin Decanoate-50, Hybolin Decanoate-100, Neo-Durabolic		
adrenocorticosteroids adrenocorticotropic hormones	May increase potential for fluid and electrolyte retention.	• Monitor serum electrolyte levels. • Monitor patient for edema.
insulin oral antidiabetics	May decrease blood glucose level.	• Monitor serum glucose level closely. • Monitor patient carefully for signs of hypoglycemia, including dizziness, diaphoresis, confusion, and tachycardia. • Dosage adjustment may be needed.
warfarin-type anticoagulants	May increase PT and INR.	• Monitor PT and INR. • Monitor patient for increased bruising or bleeding tendencies.
naproxen • Naprosyn, EC-Naprosyn **naproxen sodium** • Aleve, Anaprox, Naprelan		
acetaminophen anti-inflammatory drugs gold compounds	May increase nephrotoxicity.	• Monitor renal function test results closely.
anticoagulants	May increase anticoagulant effects.	• Monitor PT, PTT, and INR.

thrombolytics (coumarin derivatives, heparin, streptokinase, urokinase)		• Monitor patient for increased bleeding tendencies. • Dosage adjustment may be needed.
antihypertensives diuretics	May decrease effectiveness of these drugs; diuretics may increase nephrotoxicity.	• Monitor BP and renal function test results.
anti-inflammatory drugs corticosteroids corticotropin salicylates	May increase risk of adverse GI reactions, including ulceration and hemorrhage.	• Avoid using together, if possible. • If not possible, monitor patient closely. • Monitor patient for increased GI complaints, abdominal pain, and melena.
anti-inflammatory drugs aspirin parenteral carbenicillin cefamandole cefoperazone dextran dipyridamole mezlocillin piperacillin plicamycin salicylates sulfinpyrazone ticarcillin valproic acid	May increase risk of bleeding from inhibited platelet aggregation.	• Avoid using together, if possible. • If not possible, monitor patient closely. • Monitor PT and INR. • Monitor patient for increased bleeding or bruising tendencies.
aspirin	May decrease the bioavailability of naproxen.	• Monitor patient for drug effect.
coumadin derivatives nifedipine phenytoin verapamil	Toxicity of these drugs may occur.	• Monitor PT and INR and serum drug levels, as appropriate. • Assess patient for signs of drug toxicity.

(continued)

INTERACTING AGENTS	POSSIBLE EFFECTS	NURSING CONSIDERATIONS
naproxen (continued)		
insulin oral antidiabetics	May potentiate hypoglycemic effects.	• Monitor serum glucose level closely. • Monitor patient carefully for signs of hypoglycemia, including dizziness, diaphoresis, confusion, and tachycardia. • Dosage adjustment may be needed.
lithium methotrexate	May decrease renal clearance of these drugs.	• Monitor renal function. • Monitor serum levels of these drugs. • Check for signs of lithium toxicity: sedation, confusion, tremors, muscle stiffness, increased deep tendon reflexes, visual changes, nystagmus. • Check for signs of methotrexate toxicity: myelosuppression, anemia, nausea, vomiting, diarrhea, dermatitis, alopecia, melena, or fatigue.
naratriptan hydrochloride • Amerge		
ergot-containing or ergot-type drugs (or other 5-HT$_1$ agonists)	May prolong vasospastic reactions.	• Use of these drugs within 24 hr of naratriptan is contraindicated.
oral contraceptives	May increase naratriptan level.	• Monitor patient for increased adverse effects. • Dosage adjustment may be needed.
SSRIs (such as fluoxetine, fluvoxamine, paroxetine, sertraline)	May cause weakness, hyperreflexia, and incoordination.	• Use together cautiously. • Monitor patient for these adverse effects.
sibutramine	May increase risk of serotonin syndrome (altered mental status; increased muscle tone, weakness, twitching; hyperther- ~~mia; delirium; coma; death~~)	• Avoid using together.

| smoking | May increase naratriptan clearance by 30%. | • Discourage smoking. |

nefazodone hydrochloride • Serzone

alprazolam triazolam	May potentiate effects of these drugs.	• Don't administer together. • If concomitant use is needed, dosages of alprazolam and triazolam may need to be reduced greatly.
CNS-active drugs	May cause additive CNS effects.	• Use together cautiously. • Monitor patient for adverse effects, including increased sedation, dizziness, agitation, and asthenia.
digoxin	May increase serum digoxin level.	• Monitor serum digoxin level. • Monitor patient for signs of toxicity.
MAO inhibitors	May cause severe excitation, hyperpyrexia, seizures, delirium, or coma.	• Don't use drug during or within 14 days of MAO inhibitor therapy.
highly plasma protein–bound drugs	May increase risk and severity of adverse reactions.	• Monitor patient for increased adverse reactions and toxic effects.
sumatriptan	May cause serotonin syndrome (altered mental status; increased muscle tone, weakness, twitching; hyperthermia; delirium; coma; death).	• Don't use together. • If unavoidable, initiate drug at low dosages and monitor patient closely.

nelfinavir mesylate • Viracept

amiodarone ergot derivatives midazolam quinidine triazolam	May increase plasma levels of these drugs, which may increase risk for serious or life-threatening adverse events.	• These drugs shouldn't be used together.

(continued)

INTERACTING AGENTS	POSSIBLE EFFECTS	NURSING CONSIDERATIONS
nelfinavir mesylate *(continued)*		
anti-HIV protease inhibitors (such as indinavir or saquinavir)	May increase plasma levels of both drugs.	• Monitor patient for increased adverse effects and clinical effects.
carbamazepine phenobarbital phenytoin	May reduce the effectiveness of nelfinavir by decreasing nelfinavir plasma level.	• Monitor patient for clinical effect.
HMG-CoA inhibitors (such as lovastatin, simvastatin)	Nelfinavir may increase plasma levels of these drugs. May increase risk of myopathy, including rhabdomyolysis.	• Monitor patient for signs of myopathy and rhabdomyolysis (increased serum creatinine kinase level, muscle aches, weakness).
oral contraceptives	Nelfinavir may decrease plasma levels of oral contraceptives.	• Advise patient to use appropriate contraceptive measures during therapy.
drugs primarily metabolized by CYP3A, (such as dihydropyridine or calcium channel blockers)	May result in increased levels of these drugs and decreased plasma level of nelfinavir.	• If used together, closely monitor patient for increased adverse effects. • Monitor patient for nelfinavir clinical effect.
rifabutin	May increase rifabutin plasma level.	• Decrease rifabutin dose..
rifampin	May decrease nelfinavir plasma level.	• Using drugs together isn't recommended.
sildenafil	May increase adverse effects of sildenafil, including severe hypotension.	• Use together cautiously; sildenafil should be given in reduced dosages.
nevirapine • Viramune		
drugs extensively metabolized by P-450 CYP3A	Nevirapine may lower the plasma levels of these drugs.	• Monitor patient for therapeutic effects. • Dosage adjustment of these drugs may be needed.

ketoconazole	May decrease ketoconazole level.	• Avoid using together.
oral contraceptives protease inhibitors	May decrease plasma levels of these drugs.	• Monitor patient for clinical effect. • Dosage adjustment of the protease inhibitor may be needed. • Advise patient to use barrier contraception.
St. John's wort	May decrease nevirapine level.	• Advise patient against using together. • Advise patient to contact a health care professional before using an herbal preparation.

nicardipine hydrochloride • Cardene, Cardene IV, Cardene SR

cimetidine	May increase plasma level of nicardipine.	• Monitor patient for increased effects. • A lower dose of nicardipine may be needed.
cyclosporine	May increase plasma level of cyclosporine.	• Monitor serum cyclosporine level and renal function test results. • Monitor patient for toxicity.
fentanyl anesthesia	May cause severe hypotension.	• Monitor BP frequently.
grapefruit juice	May increase bioavailability of drug.	• Advise patient to avoid taking drug with grapefruit juice.
high-fat meal	May decrease bioavailability of nicardipine by 20% to 30%.	• Advise patient to take between meals, if possible.

INTERACTING AGENTS	POSSIBLE EFFECTS	NURSING CONSIDERATIONS
nicotine • Habitrol, Nicoderm, Nicotrol, Nicotrol Inhaler, Nicotrol NS, ProStep		
acetaminophen caffeine imipramine oxazepam pentazocine propranolol theophylline	Cessation of smoking may decrease induction of hepatic enzymes responsible for metabolizing certain drugs.	• Monitor patient for increased adverse effects. • Monitor serum levels if appropriate. • Dosage reduction of these drugs may be needed.
adrenergic antagonists (such as labetalol and prazosin) or adrenergic agonists (such as isoproterenol and phenylephrine)	Cessation of smoking may decrease levels of circulating catecholamines.	• Dosage adjustment of these drugs may be needed.
insulin	Cessation of smoking may increase the amount of subcutaneous insulin absorbed.	• Monitor serum glucose level. • Dosage adjustment may be needed.
propoxyphene	Cessation of smoking may increase first pass metabolism of propoxyphene.	• Monitor patient for therapeutic effect. • Dosage adjustment may be needed.
blue cohosh	May increase effects of nicotine.	• Advise patient against using together. • Advise patient to contact a health care professional before using an herbal preparation.
nifedipine • Adalat, Adalat CC, Procardia, Procardia XL		
beta blockers	May exacerbate angina, heart failure, and hypotension.	• Monitor patient's cardiac function.
cimetidine	May decrease metabolism of nifedipine.	• Monitor patient for increased nifedipine adverse effects. • Dosage adjustment may be needed.

digoxin	May increase serum digoxin level.	• Monitor serum digoxin level. • Monitor patient for toxicity (fatigue, muscle weakness, visual disturbances, nausea, vomiting, arrhythmias).
fentanyl	May cause excessive hypotension.	• Monitor vital signs and cardiac rhythm.
hypotensives	May precipitate excessive hypotension.	• Monitor BP.
phenytoin	May increase phenytoin level.	• Monitor serum phenytoin level. • Monitor patient for signs of toxicity, including drowsiness, nausea, vomiting, nystagmus, ataxia, tremor, slurred speech, hypotension, and arrhythmias.
grapefruit juice	May increase bioavailability of nifedipine.	• Advise patient to avoid taking together.

nimodipine • Nimotop

antihypertensives	May enhance hypotensive effect.	• Monitor patient's BP.
calcium channel blockers	May enhance CV effects of these drugs.	• Monitor patient for increased effects. • Dosage adjustments may be needed.
phenytoin	May increase phenytoin level.	• Monitor serum phenytoin level.
food	May decrease absorption.	• Give drug 1 hr before or 2 hr after meals.

nitrofurantoin macrocrystals • Macrobid, Macrodantin
nitrofurantoin microcrystals • Furadantin

anticholinergics	May enhance bioavailability.	• Monitor patient for adverse effects; no clinical intervention should be needed.
magnesium trisilicate antacids	May decrease nitrofurantoin absorption.	• Separate administration times.
probenecid sulfinpyrazone	May reduce renal excretion of nitrofurantoin.	• Monitor for increased toxicity and decreased clinical effect.

(continued)

Interacting agents in **bold type** indicate severe, well-documented interactions.   †Canadian

INTERACTING AGENTS	POSSIBLE EFFECTS	NURSING CONSIDERATIONS
nitrofurantoin *(continued)*		
quinolone derivatives (such as cinoxacin, ciprofloxacin, nalidixic acid, norfloxacin)	May antagonize anti-infective effects.	• Monitor patient for decreased clinical effect.
food	May enhance bioavailability of nitrofurantoin.	• Give drug with food.
nitroglycerin (glyceryl trinitrate) • Nitro-Bid, Nitrocine, Nitroquick, Nitrostat, Tridil, Nitrol, Minitran, Nitro-Derm, Nitro-Dur, Transderm-Nitro		
alcohol antihypertensives phenothiazines	May cause additive hypotensive effects.	• Monitor BP closely. • Dosage adjustment may be needed to avoid orthostatic hypotension. • Advise patient to avoid alcohol.
ergot alkaloids	May precipitate angina.	• Monitor patient for angina pain.
sildenafil	May potentiate hypotensive effects of nitrates.	• Don't use together.
nitroprusside sodium • Nipride†, Nitropress		
general anesthetics (especially enflurane and halothane)	May potentiate hypotensive effects.	• Monitor BP carefully.
antihypertensives	May potentiate antihypertensive effects of nitroprusside.	• Monitor BP carefully.
pressor drugs (such as epinephrine)	May cause an increase in BP during nitroprusside therapy.	• Monitor BP carefully.
sildenafil	May potentiate hypotensive effects of nitrates.	• Avoid use together.

norfloxacin (systemic) • Noroxin

antacids multivitamins containing divalent or trivalent cations	May interfere with absorption of norfloxacin.	• Administer separately at least 2 hr apart.
cyclosporine	May increase nephrotoxicity.	• Monitor cyclosporine level and renal function test results. • An alternative antibiotic may be used if toxicity develops.
nitrofurantoin	May antagonize antibacterial activity of norfloxacin.	• Avoid using together.
probenecid	May increase serum norfloxacin level.	• May be used together for this efffect.
warfarin	May prolong PT.	• Monitor PT and INR. • Monitor patient for increased bleeding or bruising tendencies.
xanthine derivatives (such as aminophylline and theophylline)	May increase theophylline level.	• Monitor serum theophylline level. • Signs of toxicity include tachycardia, nausea, vomiting, diarrhea, restlessness, headaches, agitation, palpitations, and arrhythmias.
food	May interfere with absorption of norfloxacin.	• Give drug 1 hr before or 2 hr after meals.
sun exposure	May cause photosensitivity reaction.	• Advise patient to use sunblock.

nortriptyline hydrochloride • Aventyl, Pamelor

centrally acting antihypertensives (such as **clonidine**, guanabenz, guanadrel, guanethidine, methyldopa, reserpine)	May decrease hypotensive effects of antihypertensives.	• Avoid using with clonidine. • When used with other drugs, monitor BP frequently, especially when therapy starts. • Alternative antihypertensives may be needed.

(continued)

Interacting agents in **bold type** indicate severe, well-documented interactions.   †Canadian

INTERACTING AGENTS	POSSIBLE EFFECTS	NURSING CONSIDERATIONS
nortriptyline hydrochloride (continued)		
atropine and other anticholinergics, including antihistamines, meperidine, phenothiazines, and antiparkinsonians	May cause oversedation, paralytic ileus, visual changes, and severe constipation.	• Use these drugs together only when needed. • Monitor patient for increased sedation or respiratory depression. • Monitor patient for GI or visual complaints. • Dosage adjustment may be needed.
barbiturates	May induce nortriptyline metabolism and decrease therapeutic efficacy. May cause additive CNS depression.	• Monitor patient for clinical effect. • Monitor patient for increased sedation or respiratory depression. • Dosage adjustment may be needed.
beta blockers cimetidine methylphenidate oral contraceptives propoxyphene	May inhibit nortriptyline metabolism, increasing its plasma level.	• Monitor for nortriptyline toxicity, including excessive anticholinergic activity (agitation, confusion, hallucinations, hyperthermia, seizures, urinary retention, pupilary dilation, dry mucous membranes) followed by increased CNS-depressant effects (decreased or absent reflexes, sedation, respiratory depression, hypotension, arrhythmias, hypothermia).
CNS depressants (including analgesics, alcohol, barbiturates, narcotics, tranquilizers, anesthetics)	May cause additive CNS effects and oversedation.	• Use together cautiously. • Monitor patient for increased sedation and respiratory depression, dizziness, agitation, and asthenia. • Advise patient to avoid alcohol.
disulfiram	May cause delirium and tachycardia.	• Observe patient closely for these adverse

ethchlorvynol		effects or other signs of psychoses.
haloperidol phenothiazines	May decrease metabolism of nortriptyline, leading to an increased serum level.	• Monitor serum nortriptyline level and patient for signs of toxicity. • Dosage adjustment may be needed.
antiarrhythmics (quinidine, disopyramide, procainamide) pimozide thyroid hormones	May increase incidence of arrhythmias and conduction defects.	• Monitor ECG closely when concurrent therapy starts.
sympathomimetics, including epinephrine, phenylephrine, and ephedrine (often found in nasal sprays)	May increase BP.	• Check BP frequently. • Monitor patient for severe hypertension.
quinolones	May cause life-threatening cardiac arrhythmias.	• Don't use together.
MAO inhibitors	Hyperpyretic crises, seizures, and death may occur.	• Don't give nortriptyline during or within 2 wk of MAO inhibitor therapy.
smoking (heavy)	May induce imipramine metabolism and decrease therapeutic efficacy.	• Discourage smoking.

ofloxacin • Floxin, Ocuflox

antacids	May interfere with GI absorption of ofloxacin, resulting in decreased serum levels.	• Give antacids at least 6 hr before or 2 hr after ofloxacin.
iron salts	May decrease ofloxacin absorption.	• Give at least 2 hr apart.
antidiabetics	May affect blood glucose levels, causing hypoglycemia or hyperglycemia.	• Monitor serum glucose level closely. • Monitor patient for signs of hypoglycemia including dizziness, diaphoresis, confusion, and tachycardia. Monitor patient for signs of hyperglycemia,

(continued)

Interacting agents in **bold type** indicate severe, well-documented interactions.   †Canadian

INTERACTING AGENTS	POSSIBLE EFFECTS	NURSING CONSIDERATIONS
ofloxacin *(continued)*		
antidiabetics *(continued)*		including fatigue, polyuria, polydipsia, weight loss, abdominal pain, altered mental status, tachycardia, hypotension, glucosuria, and ketonuria. • Dosage adjustment may be needed.
theophylline	May prolong the half-life of theophylline, elevating serum theophylline level and increasing the risk of theophylline-related adverse reactions.	• Monitor theophylline level closely. • Dosage adjustment may be needed. • Signs of toxicity include tachycardia, nausea, vomiting, diarrhea, restlessness, headaches, agitation, palpitations, and arrhythmias.
warfarin	May prolong PT and INR.	• Monitor PT and INR.
sun exposure	May cause photosensitivity reactions.	• Advise patient to take precautions.
olanzapine • Zyprexa, Zyprexa Zydis		
alcohol antihypertensives diazepam	May potentiate hypotensive effects.	• Monitor BP closely. • Advise patient to avoid alcohol.
carbamazepine omeprazole rifampin	May cause increased clearance of olanzapine because these drugs inhibit CYP1A2.	• Monitor patient for clinical effects.
fluvoxamine	May inhibit olanzapine elimination.	• Monitor patient for signs of toxicity, including drowsiness, slurred speech, hypotension, altered mental status, seizures, and dystonic reactions.

dopamine agonists levodopa	May cause antagonized effects of these drugs.	• Monitor patient for clinical effects of these drugs.
St. John's wort	Herb may reduce serum level, increasing the severity of psychotic symptoms.	• Warn against concomitant use. • If serum level is adjusted for a patient already taking St. John's wort, stopping the herb could cause these levels to rise, causing toxicity. • Advise patient to contact a health care professional before using any herbs.
nutmeg	May cause a loss of symptom control or interfere with existing therapy for psychiatric illnesses.	• Advise patient against using together. • Advise patient to contact a health care professional before using any herbs.

olsalazine sodium • Dipentum

warfarin	May increase PT.	• Monitor PT and INR.

omeprazole • Prilosec

ampicillin esters iron derivatives itraconazole ketoconazole	May cause poor bioavailability because optimal absorption of these drugs requires a low gastric pH.	• Don't use together, if possible. • If unavoidable, try giving the drug with an acidic beverage.
diazepam phenytoin propranolol theophylline warfarin	Omeprazole may increase effects of these drugs.	• Monitor patient for increased clinical effects, such as prolonged sedation or increased PT and INR. • Monitor drug serum levels if appropriate. • Monitor patient for decreased effects if omeprazole is stopped after using together.

(continued)

INTERACTING AGENTS	POSSIBLE EFFECTS	NURSING CONSIDERATIONS
omeprazole (continued)		
male fern	May inactivate drug in alkaline environments.	• Advise patient to use together cautiously. • Advise patient to consult health care provider before taking herbal preparations.
pennyroyal	May change the rate of formation of pennyroyal's toxic metabolites.	• Don't use together. • Advise patient to consult health care provider before taking herbal preparations.
ondansetron hydrochloride • Zofran, Zofran ODT		
horehound	May enhance serotonergic effects.	• Advise patient against using together. • Advise patient to consult health care provider before using any herbal preparations.
orlistat • Xenical		
fat-soluble vitamins (such as vitamin E and beta-carotene)	May decrease absorption.	• Separate administration times by 2 hr.
pravastatin	May cause slightly increased pravastatin levels and additive lipid-lowering effects of drug.	• Monitor patient for clinical effects and adverse effects. • Monitor lipid levels.
warfarin	May cause a change in coagulation effects.	• Monitor PT and INR.
oxaprozin • Daypro		
oral anticoagulants	May increase the risk of bleeding.	• Monitor PT and INR.
aspirin	Oxaprozin may displace salicylates from	• Monitor patient for signs and symptoms

	plasma protein binding, increasing the risk of salicylate toxicity.	of salicylate toxicity, including increased respiratory rate, tinnitus, vomiting, headache, irritability, and seizures.
beta blockers (such as metoprolol)	May cause a transient increase in BP after 14 days.	• Monitor BP.
methotrexate	May decrease renal clearance of methotrexate.	• Monitor patient for signs of methotrexate toxicity, including myelosuppression, anemia, nausea, vomiting, diarrhea, dermatitis, alopecia, melena, and fatigue. • Monitor serum methotrexate level.
sun exposure	May cause photosensitivity reactions.	• Advise patient to use sunblock.

oxazepam • Apo-Oxazepam†, Novoxapam†, Ox-pam†, Serax

alcohol antidepressants antihistamines barbiturates general anesthetics MAO inhibitors narcotics phenothiazines	Oxazepam may potentiate the CNS-depressant effects of these drugs.	• Monitor patient closely for increased sedation, dizziness, ataxia, tremor, agitation, or respiratory depression. • Advise patient to avoid alcohol.
antacids	May decrease the rate of oxazepam absorption.	• Separate administration times of these drugs.
cimetidine disulfiram	May diminish hepatic metabolism of oxazepam, increasing its plasma level.	• Monitor patient for increased adverse effects. • Oxazepam dosage may need to be reduced.
levodopa	May inhibit levodopa's therapeutic effects.	• Monitor patient closely for clinical effect. • Oxazepam may need to be stopped.

(continued)

Interacting agents in **bold type** indicate severe, well-documented interactions.   †Canadian

INTERACTING AGENTS	POSSIBLE EFFECTS	NURSING CONSIDERATIONS
oxazepam (continued)		
smoking (heavy)	May accelerate oxazepam metabolism, lowering clinical effectiveness.	• Monitor patient for clinical effect. • Discourage smoking.
oxcarbazepine • Trileptal		
carbamazepine valproic acid verapamil	May decrease serum level of active metabolite of oxcarbazepine.	• Monitor serum drug level closely. • Monitor patient for adequate seizure control.
felodipine	May decrease felodipine level.	• Monitor patient for adequate BP control.
hormonal contraceptives	May decrease plasma level of ethinylestradiol and levonorgestrel and reduce effectiveness of oral contraceptives.	• Women of childbearing age should use alternative forms of contraception.
phenobarbital	May decrease serum level of active metabolite of oxcarbazepine. May increase phenobarbital level.	• Monitor serum drug level closely. • Monitor patient for adequate seizure control. • Monitor patient for signs of phenobarbital toxicity, including ataxia, slurred speech, sustained nystagmus, somnolence, confusion, respiratory depression, pulmonary edema, areflexia, and coma.
phenytoin	May decrease serum level of active metabolite of oxcarbazepine. May increase phenytoin level in adults receiving high doses of oxcarbazepine.	• Monitor phenytoin level closely when therapy starts. • Check for signs of phenytoin toxicity, including drowsiness, decreased level of consciousness, nausea, vomiting, nystagmus, ataxia, dysarthria, tremor, slurred speech, hypotension, arrhythmias, and respiratory depression.

alcohol	May increase CNS depression.	• Discourage using together.

oxtriphylline • Apo-Oxtriphylline†, Choledyl, Choledyl SA

lithium	Oxtriphylline may increase lithium excretion.	• Monitor patient for clinical effect.
acyclovir allopurinol (high dose) cimetidine diltiazem macrolides (erythromycin, troleandomycin) propranolol quinolones zileuton	May increase the serum level of oxtriphylline by decreasing hepatic clearance.	• Monitor oxtriphylline level. • Signs and symptoms of toxicity include tachycardia, nausea, vomiting, diarrhea, restlessness, insomnia, irritability, headaches, agitation, palpitations, arrhythmias, tachypnea, and seizures. • Dosage adjustments may be needed; for example, when starting zileuton in patients receiving oxtriphylline, oxtriphylline dose may be reduced by 50%.
adenosine	May antagonize effects on the heart.	• Larger doses of adenosine may be required, or adenosine may be ineffective.
aminoglutethimide barbiturates	May decrease effects of oxtriphylline by enhancing its metabolism.	• Monitor patient for clinical effect.
beta blockers	May increase serum theophylline level and antagonistic pharmacologic effect of either drug.	• Monitor serum theophylline level, especially if beta blocker is added or stopped. • Monitor patient for clinical effects.
halothane	May potentiate cardiac arrhythmias.	• Don't use together.
marijuana nicotine	May decrease effects of oxtriphylline by enhancing its metabolism.	• Discourage marijuana and nicotine use.

INTERACTING AGENTS	POSSIBLE EFFECTS	NURSING CONSIDERATIONS
oxycodone hydrochloride • OxyContin, OxyFAST, Oxy IR, Roxicodone, Supeudol†		
general anesthetics	May cause severe CV depression.	• Use together with extreme caution. • Monitor patient's vital signs and ECG closely.
anticholinergics	May cause paralytic ileus.	• Use together cautiously. • Monitor patient for increased GI complaints, abdominal pain, nausea and vomiting, and absence of bowel sounds.
anticoagulants	Oxycodone products containing aspirin may increase effects of anticoagulant.	• Monitor PT and INR. • Monitor patient for increased bleeding tendencies.
alcohol CNS depressants (such as general anesthetics, antihistamines, barbiturates, benzodiazepines, muscle relaxants, narcotic analgesics, phenothiazines, sedative-hypnotics, TCAs)	May potentiate respiratory and CNS depression, sedation, and hypotensive effects of drug.	• Use together cautiously. • Monitor patient closely for increased CNS depressant effects (sedation, dizziness, ataxia, tremor, agitation, respiratory depression). • Monitor BP. • Oxycodone or other drug dose may need to be reduced. • Advise patient to avoid alcohol.
cimetidine	May increase respiratory and CNS depression, causing confusion, disorientation, apnea, or seizures.	• Avoid using together. • If drugs are used together, monitor patient for adverse CNS effects. A narcotic antagonist (such as naloxone) will reverse these effects.

digitoxin phenytoin rifampin	May cause drug accumulation and enhanced effects from use with drugs that are extensively metabolized in the liver.	• Monitor patient closely for increased adverse effects.
opioid agonist-antagonist or a single dose of an antagonist	Patient who becomes physically dependent on oxycodone may experience acute withdrawal syndrome.	• Use together cautiously. • Signs of withdrawal include restlessness, lacrimation, rhinorrhea, yawning, diaphoresis, chills, myalgias, mydriasis, abdominal cramps, nausea, vomiting, diarrhea, and increased respiratory rate, HR, or BP.

oxymorphone hydrochloride • Numorphan

general anesthetics	May cause severe CV depression.	• Monitor vital signs and ECG closely.
anticholinergics	May cause paralytic ileus.	• Monitor patient for abdominal pain, distension, decreased or absent bowel sounds, nausea, or vomiting.
cimetidine	May increase respiratory and CNS depression, causing confusion, disorientation, apnea, or seizures.	• Monitor patient's respiratory status. • Dosage of meperidine may need to be reduced or one or both drugs stopped. • Be prepared to give a narcotic antagonist.
alcohol CNS depressants (such as general anesthetics, antihistamines, barbiturates, benzodiazepines, muscle relaxants, opiates, phenothiazines, sedative-hypnotics, TCAs)	May potentiate respiratory and CNS depression, sedation, and hypotensive effects of drug.	• Use together cautiously. • Monitor patient closely for increased sedation, dizziness, ataxia, tremor, agitation, respiratory depression, and hypotension. • Dosage adjustment may be needed. • Advise patient to avoid alcohol.

(continued)

Interacting agents in **bold type** indicate severe, well-documented interactions.   †Canadian

INTERACTING AGENTS	POSSIBLE EFFECTS	NURSING CONSIDERATIONS
oxymorphone hydrochloride *(continued)*		
digitoxin phenytoin rifampin	May cause drug accumulation and enhanced effects from use with other drugs that are extensively metabolized in the liver.	• Monitor patient for increased serum level. • Check for signs of toxicity. • Dosage adjustments may be needed.
opioid agonist-antagonist or a single dose of an antagonist	May cause acute withdrawal syndrome in patients who become physically dependent on oxymorphone.	• Avoid use together unless indicated.
paclitaxel • Taxol		
cisplatin	Myelosuppression may be greater when cisplatin is given before, rather than after, paclitaxel.	• Consider this effect before therapy.
cyclosporine dexamethasone diazepam etoposide ketoconazole quinidine teniposide verapamil vincristine	May inhibit paclitaxel metabolism.	• Monitor patient for signs of toxicity, including increased bone marrow suppression, peripheral neurotoxicity, and mucositis. • Dosage reduction may be needed.
pancreatin • Donnazyme, Hi-Vegi-Lip, 4X Pancreatin, 8X Pancreatin, Pancrezyme 4X		
antacids containing calcium or magnesium	May reduce pancreatin activity.	• Separate administration times.
iron products	May decrease absorption of these drugs.	• Separate administration times. • Monitor patient for decreased effectiveness.

pancrelipase • Cotazym, Cotazym-S, Creon 5, Creon 10, Creon 20, Ilozyme, Ku-Zyme HP, Pancrease, Pancrease MT4, Pancrease MT10, Pancrease MT16, Pancrease MT20, Ultrase, Ultrase MT12, Ultrase MT18, Ultrase MT20, Viokase, Zymase

antacids containing calcium or magnesium	May reduce pancrelipase activity.	• Separate administration times.
iron products	May decrease absorption of these drugs.	• Separate administration times. • Monitor patient for decreased effectiveness.

pantoprazole • Protonix

ampicillin esters ketoconazole iron salts	May decrease or increase absorption of these drugs.	• Monitor patient for clinical effects or toxicity. • Dosage adjustments may be needed.
food	May delay absorption of pantoprazole for up to 2 hr; however, the extent of absorption is not affected.	• Drug can be given without regard to meals.

paricalcitol • Zemplar

digoxin	Hypercalcemia may worsen digitalis toxicity.	• Monitor serum calcium and digoxin levels.

paroxetine hydrochloride • Paxil

cimetidine	May decrease hepatic metabolism of paroxetine; increases risk of toxicity.	• Dosage adjustments of paroxetine may be needed.
digoxin	May decrease digoxin level.	• Monitor patient for clinical effect. • Monitor serum digoxin level.
MAO inhibitors	May increase risk of serious, sometimes fatal, adverse reactions.	• Don't use paroxetine during or within 14 days of MAO inhibitor therapy.

(continued)

INTERACTING AGENTS	POSSIBLE EFFECTS	NURSING CONSIDERATIONS
paroxetine hydrochloride (continued)		
phenobarbital	May induce paroxetine metabolism. May reduce plasma level of drug.	• Dosage adjustment may be needed.
phenytoin	May alter pharmacokinetics of phenytoin.	• Monitor serum phenytoin level. • Dosage adjustment may be needed.
procyclidine	May increase procyclidine level.	• Monitor patient for excessive anti-cholinergic effects.
theophylline	May increase theophylline level.	• Monitor theophylline level closely. • Dosage adjustment may be needed. • Signs of toxicity include tachycardia, nausea, vomiting, diarrhea, restlessness, headaches, agitation, palpitations, and arrhythmias.
tryptophan	May increase adverse reactions, such as diaphoresis, headache, nausea, and dizziness.	• Use together cautiously. • Monitor patient for increased adverse effects.
warfarin	May increase risk of bleeding.	• Monitor PT and INR.
sibutramine sumatriptan sympathomimetics	May increase risk of serotonin syndrome (altered mental status; increased muscle tone, weakness, twitching; hyperthermia; delirium; coma; death).	• Avoid using with sympathomimetics, sibutramine, or sumatriptan, if possible. • Monitor patient for increased CNS effects.
St. John's wort	May cause sedative-hypnotic intoxication.	• Advise patient to avoid using together. • Advise patient to consult health care provider before taking herbal preparations.
alcohol	May increase risk of CNS adverse effects.	• Discourage concomitant use.

pemoline • Cylert

anticonvulsants	May decrease seizure threshold.	• Monitor patient for loss of seizure control.
caffeine	May decrease efficacy of pemoline in attention-deficit hyperactivity disorder.	• Discourage use together.

penbutolol sulfate • Levatol

clonidine	May cause paradoxical hypertension when combined with beta blockers. May enhance rebound hypertension when clonidine is withdrawn.	• Monitor BP when either drug is started or withdrawn during concomitant therapy. • If discontinuing these drugs, penbutolol should be stopped first.
doxazosin prazosin terazosin	May enhance first-dose orthostatic hypotension with these drugs.	• Monitor BP closely with first dose. • Take safety precautions.
insulin oral antidiabetics	May alter hypoglycemic response. Effects of sulfonylureas may be decreased.	• Monitor serum glucose level. • Monitor patient for signs of hyperglycemia (fatigue, polyuria, polydipsia, weight loss, abdominal pain, altered mental status, tachycardia, hypotension, glucosuria, ketonuria) or hypoglycemia, including dizziness, diaphoresis, confusion, and tachycardia.
epinephrine	May cause hypertensive episode followed by bradycardia.	• Penbutolol should be stopped 3 days before anticipated epinephrine use. • Don't use together. • Monitor BP.

(continued)

Interacting agents in **bold type** indicate severe, well-documented interactions.   †Canadian

INTERACTING AGENTS	POSSIBLE EFFECTS	NURSING CONSIDERATIONS
penbutolol sulfate (continued)		
ergot alkaloids	May increase potential for peripheral ischemia or gangrene.	• Monitor patient for peripheral ischemia (cold extremities); dosage adjustment or withdrawal of drug may be needed.
lidocaine	May increase volume of distribution of lidocaine; may increase loading dose requirements in some patients.	• Monitor patient for clinical effects. • Dosage increase may be needed.
indomethacin NSAIDs	May antagonize antihypertensive effects of atenolol.	• Avoid using together, if possible. • Monitor BP; dosage adjustment may be needed.
oral calcium antagonists	May enhance hypotensive effects of beta blockers and predispose patient to bradycardia and arrhythmias.	• Monitor cardiac function. • Dosage adjustment may be needed.
reserpine catecholamine-depleting drugs	May cause additive effects.	• Monitor BP and HR closely.
theophylline	May increase serum theophylline levels. May decrease effects of both drugs.	• Monitor serum theophylline level. • Monitor patient for signs of toxicity, including tachycardia, nausea, vomiting, diarrhea, restlessness, headaches, agitation, palpitations, arrhythmias, and seizures. • Dosage adjustment may be needed.

penicillin G benzathine • Bicillin L-A, Permapen
penicillin G benzathine and procaine • Bicillin C-R
penicillin G potassium • Pfizerpen
penicillin G procaine • Ayercillin†, Bicillin C-R, Wycillin
penicillin G sodium

aminoglycosides	May cause synergistic therapeutic effects, chiefly against enterococci; combination is most effective against enterococcal bacterial endocarditis. Drugs are physically and chemically incompatible; inactivated when mixed or given together.	• Give drugs separately.
heparin oral anticoagulants	May increase risk of bleeding.	• Monitor PTT, PT, and INR. • Monitor patient for increased bleeding tendencies.
methotrexate	Large doses of penicillin may interfere with renal tubular secretion of methotrexate; may delay elimination and elevate serum level of methotrexate.	• Monitor serum methotrexate level. • Signs of toxicity include myelosuppression, anemia, nausea, vomiting, diarrhea, dermatitis, alopecia, melena, and fatigue.
NSAIDs sulfinpyrazone	May prolong penicillin half-life.	• Monitor patient for clinical effectiveness.
oral contraceptives	May decrease contraceptive effectiveness.	• Advise patient to use barrier contraception.
potassium-sparing diuretics	May cause hyperkalemia when used with parenteral penicillin G potassium.	• Monitor renal function and serum potassium level. • Monitor patient for hyperkalemia. Advise patient to avoid using potassium salt substitutes.
probenecid	May block tubular secretion of penicillin, raising its serum levels.	• Probenecid may be used for this clinical effect.
tetracyclines	May reduce penicillin effectiveness.	• Don't use together.

Interacting agents in **bold type** indicate severe, well-documented interactions.   †Canadian

INTERACTING AGENTS	POSSIBLE EFFECTS	NURSING CONSIDERATIONS
pentamidine isethionate • NebuPent, Pentacarinat, Pentam 300		
aminoglycosides amphotericin B capreomycin cisplatin colistin methoxyflurane polymyxin B vancomycin	May cause additive nephrotoxic effects.	• Avoid use together, if possible. • If used together, monitor serum levels and monitor renal function test results. • Dosage adjustments or alternative drugs may be needed.
pentobarbital sodium • Nembutal		
alcohol antidepressants antihistamines narcotics sedative-hypnotics tranquilizers	May potentiate or add CNS- and respiratory-depressant effects.	• Use together cautiously. • Monitor patient for increased sedation, dizziness, agitation, asthenia, and respiratory depression. • Advise patient to avoid alcohol.
corticosteroids digitoxin doxycycline oral contraceptives (and other estrogens) theophylline (and other xanthines)	May enhance hepatic metabolism of these drugs.	• Monitor patient for clinical effectiveness. • Monitor serum drug levels if appropriate. • Advise patient to use barrier contraception.
disulfiram MAO inhibitors valproic acid	May decrease metabolism of pentobarbital.	• Monitor serum levels closely. • Monitor patient for adequate seizure control. • Monitor patient for signs of phenobarbital toxicity, including ataxia, slurred speech, sustained nystagmus, somnolence, confusion, respiratory depression,

pulmonary edema, areflexia, and coma.

griseofulvin	May impair effectiveness of this drug. May decrease absorption from GI tract.	• Separate administration times. • Dosage adjustment may be needed.
rifampin	May decrease pentobarbital level. May increase hepatic metabolism.	• Monitor patient for clinical effects. • Dosage adjustment may be needed.
warfarin **oral anticoagulants**	May enhance enzymatic degradation of these drugs.	• Increased doses of anticoagulants may be needed. • Monitor PT and INR.

pergolide mesylate • Permax

dopamine antagonists (such as butyrophe- nones, phenothiazines, thioxanthenes) metoclopramide	May antagonize effects of pergolide.	• Avoid use together.
drugs known to affect protein binding	Pergolide is 90% protein-bound and may compete for binding sites, affecting circulating plasma levels.	• Use together cautiously. • Monitor patient for clinical effects of drugs. • Monitor patient for signs of toxicity..

perphenazine • Apo-Perphenazine†, Trilafon

antacids containing aluminum and magnesium antidiarrheals	May inhibit absorption.	• Separate administration times by at least 2 hr.
antiarrhythmics disopyramide procainamide quinidine quinolones (sparfloxacin)	May increase risk of arrhythmias and conduction defects.	• Use together cautiously. • Monitor vital signs and ECG closely. • Don't use sparfloxacin with perphenazine.

(continued)

INTERACTING AGENTS	POSSIBLE EFFECTS	NURSING CONSIDERATIONS
perphenazine *(continued)*		
appetite suppressants sympathomimetics (such as ephedrine [commonly found in nasal sprays], epinephrine, phenylephrine)	May decrease stimulatory and pressor effects; may cause epinephrine reversal (hypotensive response to epinephrine).	• Monitor patient for clinical effect. • Advise patient not to take appetite suppressants. • Epinephrine shouldn't be used in an emergent situation (such as severe hypotension) because perphenazine may block the vasopressor effects.
atropine anticholinergics (such as antidepressants, antihistamines, antiparkinsonians, MAO inhibitors, meperidine, phenothiazines)	May cause oversedation, paralytic ileus, visual changes, and severe constipation.	• Use together only when needed. • Monitor patient closely for adverse effects. • Dosage adjustment or withdrawal of drugs may be needed.
beta blockers	May inhibit perphenazine metabolism and increase plasma level and toxicity.	• Monitor patient for signs of toxicity, including deep unarousable sleep with potential coma, hypotension or hypertension, extrapyramidal symptoms, dystonia, abnormal involuntary muscle movements, agitation, seizures, arrhythmias, hypothermia or hyperthermia, and autonomic nervous dysfunction. • Dosage adjustment may be needed.
bromocriptine	May antagonize prolactin secretion.	• Avoid using together, if possible. • If used together, monitor patient for clinical effect. • Bromocriptine dose may need to be increased.

centrally acting antihypertensives (such as clonidine, guanabenz, guanadrel, guanethidine, methyldopa, reserpine)	May inhibit BP response.	• Monitor BP carefully. • Dosage may need to be adjusted or drugs stopped.
alcohol CNS depressants (such as analgesics; barbiturates; epidural, general, spinal anesthetics; narcotics; tranquilizers)	May cause oversedation, respiratory depression, and hypotension.	• Monitor patient closely for signs of increased CNS depression, including increased sedation, headache, dizziness, ataxia, confusion, agitation, respiratory depression, and hypotension. • Advise patient to avoid alcohol.
high-dose dopamine	May decrease vasoconstricting effects.	• Monitor patient closely for clinical response.
levodopa	May decrease effectiveness. May increase risk of levodopa toxicity.	• Monitor patient for clinical response to levodopa and toxicity.
lithium	May cause severe neurologic toxicity with encephalitis-like syndrome. May decrease therapeutic response to perphenazine.	• Monitor patient very closely. • Monitor patient for signs of toxicity, including sedation, confusion, tremors, muscle stiffness, increased deep tendon reflexes, visual changes, and nystagmus. • Dosage adjustment or withdrawal of drugs may be needed.
metrizamide	May increase risk of seizures.	• Monitor patient closely for increased seizures.
nitrates	May cause hypotension.	• Monitor BP.
phenobarbital	May enhance renal excretion of perphenazine.	• Dosage adjustment may be needed.
phenytoin	May inhibit metabolism and increase risk of phenytoin toxicity.	• Monitor serum phenytoin level. • Check for signs of phenytoin toxicity, including drowsiness, confusion, or de-

(continued)

INTERACTING AGENTS	POSSIBLE EFFECTS	NURSING CONSIDERATIONS
perphenazine *(continued)*		
phenytoin *(continued)*		creased level of consciousness, nausea, vomiting, nystagmus, ataxia, dysarthria, tremor, slurred speech, hypotension, arrhythmias, and respiratory depression.
propylthiouracil	May increase risk of agranulocytosis.	• Monitor hematologic studies.
yohimbe	Yohimbe is a relatively toxic herb. Perphenazine may increase the risk of herb toxicity.	• Discourage concomitant use. • Advise patient to contact health care professional before using herbs.
kava	May increase the risk or severity of dystonic reactions.	• Discourage concomitant use.
caffeine	May decrease therapeutic response to perphenazine.	• Discourage use.
smoking (heavy)	May decrease therapeutic response to perphenazine.	• Discourage smoking.
sun exposure	May cause photosensitivity reactions.	• Advise patient to use sunblock.
phenobarbital • Barbita, Solfoton **phenobarbital sodium** • Luminal		
alcohol antidepressants antihistamines narcotics sedative-hypnotics tranquilizers	May potentiate or increase CNS- and respiratory-depressant effects.	• Use together cautiously. • Monitor patient for increased sedation, dizziness, agitation, asthenia, and respiratory depression. • Advise patient to avoid alcohol.

corticosteroids digitoxin doxycycline oral contraceptives (and other estrogens) theophylline (and other xanthines)	May enhance hepatic metabolism of these drugs.	• Monitor patient for clinical effectiveness. • Monitor serum drug levels if appropriate. • Advise patient to use barrier contraception.
disulfiram MAO inhibitors valproic acid	May decrease metabolism of phenobarbital and increase toxicity.	• Monitor serum level closely. • Monitor patient for adequate seizure control. • Monitor patient for signs of phenobarbital toxicity, including ataxia, slurred speech, sustained nystagmus, somnolence, confusion, respiratory depression, pulmonary edema, areflexia, and coma.
griseofulvin	May decrease absorption from GI tract.	• Separate administration times by at least 2 hr.
rifampin	May decrease phenobarbital level because of increased hepatic metabolism.	• Monitor patient for clinical effects. • Dosage adjustment may be needed.
oral anticoagulants **warfarin**	May enhance enzymatic degradation of these drugs.	• Increased doses of anticoagulants may be needed. • Monitor PT and INR.

phentermine hydrochloride • Adipex-P, Fastin, Ionamin, Obe-Nix, Phentride, Teramine

acetazolamide antacids sodium bicarbonate	May increase renal reabsorption of phentermine and prolong duration of action.	• Monitor patient closely for increased adverse effects.
general anesthetics	May induce arrhythmias.	• Monitor vital signs and ECG closely.

(continued)

INTERACTING AGENTS	POSSIBLE EFFECTS	NURSING CONSIDERATIONS
phentermine hydrochloride *(continued)*		
antihypertensives guanethidine	May decrease hypotensive effects.	• Monitor BP.
haloperidol phenothiazines	May decrease phentermine effects.	• Monitor patient for clinical effect.
insulin	May alter insulin requirements in diabetic patient.	• Monitor serum glucose level.
sympathomimetics	May increase risk of serotonin syndrome (altered mental status; increased muscle tone, weakness, twitching; hyperthermia; delirium; coma; death).	• Don't use with sympathomimetics, if possible. • Monitor patient for increased CNS effects.
MAO inhibitors	Using together or within 14 days may cause hypertensive crisis.	• Don't use together.
caffeine	May cause additive CNS stimulation.	• Discourage excessive use.
phentolamine mesylate • Regitine		
ephedrine epinephrine	May antagonize vasoconstrictor and hypertensive effects of these drugs.	• Avoid using together
phenylephrine hydrochloride (nasal) • Alconefrin 12, Alconefrin 25, Neo-Synephrine, Nostril, Rhinall, Sinex **phenylephrine hydrochloride (parenteral)** • Neo-Synephrine **phenylephrine hydrochloride (ophthalmic)** • AK-Dilate, AK-Nefrin, Isopto Frin, Mydfrin, Neo-Synephrine, Prefrin Liquifilm		
alpha blockers antihypertensives diuretics used as antihypertensives guanadrel guanethidine	May decrease pressor response (hypotension).	• Avoid use together, if possible; alternative therapies should be used. • If necessary to use together, monitor BP. • Monitor patient closely for expected clinical effects.

nitrates
rauwolfia alkaloids

cardiac glycosides epinephrine general anesthetics (cyclopropane, halothane) guanadrel guanethidine levodopa **MAO inhibitors** TCAs sympathomimetics	May increase risk of arrhythmias, including tachycardia.	• Don't give with other sympathomimetic drugs, guanadrel, guanethidine, general anesthetics, cardiac glycosides, levodopa, and TCAs, if possible. • If used together, monitor patient closely; monitor ECG for arrhythmias and vital signs. • Allow 14 days after stopping MAO inhibitor before using phenylephrine.
cycloplegic antimuscarinics (such as atropine)	May increase mydriatic response to phenylephrine.	• May be used concomitantly for this clinical effect.
doxapram ergot alkaloids furazolidone **MAO inhibitors** mazindol methyldopa oxytocics	May potentiate pressor effects.	• Monitor patient for adverse effects, such as tachycardia, arrhythmias, hypertension, and headache. • Allow 14 days to lapse after stopping MAO inhibitor before using phenylephrine. • Dosage adjustment may be needed.
levodopa	May decrease mydriatic response to phenylephrine.	• Avoid use together, if possible. • If used together, an increased dose may be needed.
nitrates	May reduce antianginal effects.	• Evaluate response to therapy.
thyroid hormones	May increase effects of either drug.	• Monitor ECG and vital signs closely. • Monitor patient for increased adverse effects.

INTERACTING AGENTS	POSSIBLE EFFECTS	NURSING CONSIDERATIONS

phenytoin, phenytoin sodium, phenytoin sodium (extended) • Dilantin, Dilantin Infatab, Dilantin Kapseals, Dilantin-125
phenytoin sodium (prompt)

INTERACTING AGENTS	POSSIBLE EFFECTS	NURSING CONSIDERATIONS
allopurinol amiodarone benzodiazepines chloramphenicol chlorpheniramine cimetidine diazepam disulfiram **fluconazole** fluoxetine gabapentin ibuprofen imipramine isoniazid methylphenidate metronidazole miconazole nifedipine omeprazole phenacemide phenylbutazone salicylates sertraline succinimides trimethoprim valproic acid	May increase serum level of phenytoin.	• Monitor serum phenytoin level. • Monitor patient for signs of phenytoin toxicity, including drowsiness, confusion or decreased level of consciousness, nausea, vomiting, nystagmus, ataxia, dysarthia, tremor, slurred speech, hypotension, arrhythmias, and respiratory depression. • Monitor serum phenytoin level if any of these drugs are stopped while patient is still taking phenytoin. • Dosage adjustments may be needed.

acetaminophen	May decrease effects of these drugs via increased hepatic metabolism.	• Use together cautiously.
amiodarone		• Monitor patient for expected clinical effects; e.g., if phenytoin is given during a dopamine infusion, severe hypotension, and possibly cardiac arrest may occur; monitor BP closely.
benzodiazepines		
carbamazepine		
corticosteroids		
cyclosporine		
dicumarol		• Monitor therapeutic drug levels of these drugs if appropriate.
digoxin		
disopyramide		• Dosage adjustments may be needed.
dopamine		• Advise patient to use barrier contraception.
doxycycline		
estrogens		
furosemide		
haloperidol		
levodopa		
mebendazole		
meperidine		
methadone		
metyrapone		
oral contraceptives		
phenothiazines		
quinidine		
sulfonylureas		

alcohol	May decrease therapeutic effects of phenytoin.	• Monitor patient closely for clinical effectiveness of phenytoin therapy.
antacids		• Monitor patient for adequate and previously attained seizure control.
antineoplastics		
barbiturates		• Monitor serum phenytoin level.
calcium		• Dosage adjustments may be needed.
calcium gluconate		• Separate antacid and phenytoin administration times.
carbamazepine		
charcoal		• Monitor patient for toxicity if one of
diazoxide		

(continued)

INTERACTING AGENTS	POSSIBLE EFFECTS	NURSING CONSIDERATIONS
phenytoin, phenytoin sodium, phenytoin sodium (extended), phenytoin sodium (prompt) *(continued)*		
folic acid loxapine nitrofurantoin pyridoxine quinolones rifampin sucralfate theophylline		these drugs is stopped while patient is still taking phenytoin. • Advise patient to avoid alcohol.
antipsychotics	May lower seizure threshold.	• Use together cautiously. • Monitor patient for adequate and previously attained seizure control.
anticoagulants	May increase serum phenytoin level and risk of bleeding.	• Monitor serum phenytoin level. • Monitor PT and INR.
physostigmine salicylate • Antilirium **physostigmine sulfate** • Eserine		
succinylcholine	May prolong respiratory depression from inhibition of succinylcholine hydrolysis by plasma esterases.	• Monitor patient's respiratory status closely. • Monitor patient for return of spontaneous muscle activity and spontaneous respiration.
systemic cholinergics	May cause additive toxicity.	• Monitor patient for signs of toxicity, including headache, nausea, vomiting, diarrhea, blurred vision, miosis, myopia, excessive tearing, bronchospasm, hypotension, incoordination, excessive sweating, muscle weakness, bradycardia, excessive salivation, restlessness,

		agitation, and confusion.
jaborandi tree pill-bearing spurge	May cause additive effects.	• Advise patient against using together. • Advise patient to contact health care professional before using any herbal preparations.

pimozide • Orap

amphetamines methylphenidate pemoline	May cause Tourette-like tic and exacerbate existing tics.	• Don't use together; these drugs should be stopped before pimozide therapy.
azole antifungals macrolide antibiotics nefazodone protease inhibitors	These drugs may inhibit the CYP3A enzyme system and impede the metabolism of pimozide	• Use together is contraindicated.
anticonvulsants (carbamazepine, phenobarbital, phenytoin)	May lower the seizure threshold.	• Anticonvulsant dosage increase may be needed.
antiarrhythmics antidepressants antipsychotics disopyramide macrolide antibiotics phenothiazines procainamide quinidine	May further depress cardiac conduction and prolong QT interval, resulting in serious arrhythmias.	• Use together is contraindicated. • If it is necessary to use these drugs together, monitor vital signs and ECG closely.
alcohol CNS depressants (such as analgesics; anxiolytics; barbiturates; epidural, general, spinal anesthetics; narcotics; tranquilizers)	May cause oversedation and respiratory depression from additive CNS-depressant effects.	• Use together cautiously. • Monitor patient for increased sedation, dizziness, agitation, asthenia, and respiratory depression. • Advise patient to avoid alcohol.

INTERACTING AGENTS	POSSIBLE EFFECTS	NURSING CONSIDERATIONS
pindolol • Visken		
antihypertensives	May potentiate antihypertensive effects.	• Monitor BP.
aminophylline theophylline	May cause mutual inhibition of therapeutic effects and may decrease theophylline clearance, especially in patients with increased theophylline clearance induced by smoking.	• Carefully monitor patient to prevent toxic accumulation of theophylline. • Monitor serum theophylline level.
clonidine	May cause life-threatening hypertension.	• Monitor BP closely during concomitant use and after one drug is stopped.
NSAIDs	Antihypertensive effects may be antagonized.	• Avoid using together, if possible. • Monitor BP. • Dosage adjustment may be needed.
verapamil	May cause additive effects.	• Don't use together, if possible. • Monitor cardiac function. • Dosage adjustments may be needed.
epinephrine	May cause hypertensive episode followed by bradycardia.	• The beta blocker should be stopped 3 days before anticipated epinephrine use. • Don't use together. • Monitor BP.
pioglitazone hydrochloride • Actos		
ketoconazole	May inhibit metabolism of pioglitazone.	• Monitor serum glucose level more frequently.
aloe bitter melon bilberry leaf burdock	May improve serum glucose control, requiring a reduction of antidiabetics.	• Advise patient to contact health care professional before using any herbal preparations. • Monitor serum glucose level.

dandelion
fenugreek
garlic
ginseng

oral contraceptives	May decrease contraceptive effectiveness.	• Advise patient to use barrier contraception.

piperacillin sodium • Pipracil

aminoglycoside antibiotics	May cause synergistic bactericidal effects against *Pseudomonas aeruginosa*, *Escherichia coli*, *Klebsiella*, *Citrobacter*, *Enterobacter*, *Serratia*, and *Proteus mirabilis*. However, drugs are physically and chemically incompatible and inactivated when mixed or given together.	• Give these drugs separately.
clavulanic acid sulbactam tazobactam	May cause synergistic bactericidal effects against certain beta-lactamase–producing bacteria.	• May be used together for this effect.
methotrexate	Large doses of penicillin may interfere with renal tubular secretion of methotrexate and cause delayed elimination and elevated serum level of methotrexate.	• Monitor serum methotrexate level. • Monitor patient for signs of toxicity, including myelosuppression, anemia, nausea, vomiting, diarrhea, dermatitis, alopecia, melena, and fatigue.
oral contraceptives	May decrease efficacy.	• Advise patient to use barrier contraception.
probenecid	May block tubular secretion of piperacillin, raising serum level of drug.	• Probenecid may be used for this purpose.
tetracyclines	May reduce penicillin effectiveness.	• Avoid using together.
vecuronium	May prolong neuromuscular blockade.	• Monitor patient's postoperative neuromuscular and respiratory function.

Interacting agents in **bold type** indicate severe, well-documented interactions.   †Canadian

INTERACTING AGENTS	POSSIBLE EFFECTS	NURSING CONSIDERATIONS
piroxicam • Apo-Piroxicam†, Feldene, Novo-Pirocam†		
acetaminophen anti-inflammatory drugs gold compounds	May increase nephrotoxicity.	• Monitor renal function test results closely.
anticoagulants thrombolytics (coumarin derivatives, he- parin, other highly protein-bound drugs)	May potentiate anticoagulant effects.	• Monitor PTT, PT, and INR.
antihypertensives diuretics	May decrease effectiveness of these drugs. Using piroxicam with diuretics may in- crease risk of nephrotoxicity.	• Monitor BP and renal function studies. • Monitor patient for signs of increased bruising or bleeding.
alcohol anti-inflammatory drugs corticosteroids corticotropin salicylates	May cause adverse GI effects, including ul- ceration and hemorrhage.	• Don't use together, if possible. • If used together, monitor patient very closely. • Monitor patient for increased GI com- plaints, abdominal pain, and melena. • Advise patient to avoid alcohol.
aspirin	May decrease bioavailability of piroxicam.	• Don't use together, if possible.
beta blockers	May decrease antihypertensive effect.	• Don't use together, if possible. • If used together, monitor BP. • Dosage adjustment may be needed.
coumarin derivatives nifedipine phenytoin verapamil	Piroxicam may displace highly protein- bound drugs.	• Monitor PT, INR, and serum drug levels, if appropriate. • Monitor patient for signs of drug toxicity.
drugs that inhibit platelet aggregation (such as aspirin, cefamandole, cefopera- zone, dextran, dipyridamole, mezlocillin,	May cause bleeding problems.	• Avoid using together, if possible. • If used together, monitor patient closely.

piperacillin, plicamycin, salicylates, sulfinpyrazone, ticarcillin, valproic acid, other anti-inflammatory drugs)		• Monitor patient for increased GI complaints, abdominal pain, melena, and also for increased bleeding or bruising tendencies.
lithium methotrexate	May decrease renal clearance of these drugs.	• Monitor patient for signs of lithium toxicity (sedation, confusion, tremors, muscle stiffness, increased deep tendon reflexes, visual changes, nystagmus). • Monitor patient for signs of methotrexate toxicity (myelosuppression, anemia, nausea, vomiting, diarrhea, dermatitis, alopecia, melena, fatigue). • Monitor serum levels of these drugs.
sun exposure	May cause photosensitivity reaction.	• Advise patient to use sunblock.

potassium chloride • Apo-K†, Cena-K, Gen-K, K-8, K-10†, Kalium Durules†, Kaochlor S-F, Kaon-Cl, Kaon-Cl-10, Kato, Kay Ciel, K+ Care, KCL†, K-Dur, K-Ide, K-Lease, K-Long†, K-Lor, Klor-Con, Klorvess, Klotrix, K-Lyte/Cl Powder, K-Med 900†, K-Norm, K-Sol, K-Tab, Micro-K Extencaps, Micro-K 10 Extencaps, Potasalan, Rum-K, Slow-K, Ten-K

ACE inhibitors (such as captopril) **potassium-sparing diuretics** potassium-containing salt substitutes	May cause severe hyperkalemia.	• Monitor serum potassium level and renal function test results. • Monitor patient for signs of hyperkalemia, including mental confusion, neuromuscular excitability, weakness, paresthesia, ascending flaccid paralysis, and cardiac abnormalities (peaked T waves, depressed ST segment, absence of P wave, prolonged QT interval, and widened QRS complex). • Advise patient to avoid salt substitutes containing potassium.

(continued)

INTERACTING AGENTS	POSSIBLE EFFECTS	NURSING CONSIDERATIONS
potassium chloride (continued)		
anticholinergics that slow GI motility	May increase chance of GI irritation and ulceration.	• Use together cautiously. • Monitor patient for increased GI complaints, abdominal pain, and melena.
digoxin	May cause arrhythmias.	• Potassium isn't recommended in digitalized patients with severe or complete heart block. • Monitor ECG
potassium products	May cause hyperkalemia within 1 to 2 days.	• Monitor serum potassium level and renal function test results.
pramipexole hydrochloride • Mirapex		
cimetidine diltiazem quinidine quinine ranitidine triamterene verapamil	May decrease clearance of pramipexole.	• Dosage adjustment of pramipexole may be needed. • Monitor patient for signs of toxicity, including increased CNS stimulation.
dopamine antagonists (butyrophenones, metoclopramide, phenothiazines, thiothixenes)	May diminish effectiveness of pramipexole.	• Don't use together.
levodopa	May increase levodopa level.	• Dosage adjustment of levodopa may be needed.
pravastatin sodium • Pravachol		
cholestyramine colestipol	May decrease plasma level of pravastatin.	• Give pravastatin 1 hr before or 4 hr after these drugs.

cimetidine ketoconazole spironolactone	May increase risk of endocrine dysfunction. May diminish the levels or activity of steroid hormones.	• No intervention appears needed. • Take complete drug history if patient develops endocrine dysfunction.

erythromycin
fibric acid derivatives (clofibrate, gemfi-
   brozil)
immunosuppressants
high doses of niacin (≥ 1 g nicotinic acid
   daily)
	May increase risk of rhabdomyolysis.	• Don't use together, if possible.
		• Monitor patient for signs of myopathy and rhabdomyolysis (increased serum creatinine kinase level, muscle aches, weakness).

chronic alcohol abuse hepatotoxic drugs	May increase risk of hepatotoxicity.	• Monitor liver function test results. • Check for signs of hepatotoxicity (jaundice, fever, abdominal pain, clay-colored stools, tea-colored urine).
gemfibrozil	May decrease protein-binding and urinary clearance of pravastatin.	• Avoid use together.
sun exposure	May cause photosensitivity reaction.	• Advise patient to use sunblock.

prazosin hydrochloride • Minipress

antihypertensives diuretics	May increase hypotensive effects.	• Monitor BP regularly.
highly protein-bound drugs	Prazosin is highly bound to plasma proteins and may interact with these drugs.	• Monitor patient closely for clinical effects and signs of toxicity.
butcher's broom	May reduce effects of drug.	• Advise patient against using together. • Advise patient to contact health care professional before using any herbal preparations.

INTERACTING AGENTS	POSSIBLE EFFECTS	NURSING CONSIDERATIONS
prednisone • Apo-Prednisone†, Deltasone, Meticorten, Orasone, Prednicen-M, Sterapred, Winpred†		
amphotericin B diuretics	May enhance hypokalemia.	• Monitor serum potassium level. • Monitor patient for signs of hypo-kalemia, including muscle weakness, fatigue, nausea, vomiting, constipation, respiratory depression, and arrhythmias.
antacids cholestyramine colestipol	May decrease prednisone absorption, decreasing prednisone's effect.	• Separate administration times.
anticholinesterase	May antagonize effects of anti-cholinesterases used in myasthenia gravis with resulting profound muscle weakness.	• Corticosteroids may have therapeutic benefits in these patients. • Monitor patient closely and have life support readily available.
oral anticoagulants	May decrease effectiveness.	• Monitor PT and INR.
barbiturates phenytoin **rifampin**	May cause decreased corticosteroid effects because of increased hepatic metabolism.	• Don't use together, if possible. • If unavoidable, monitor patient for loss of therapeutic effects. • The corticosteroid dosage may need to be increased.
cardiac glycosides	Possible hypokalemia may increase risk of toxicity.	• Monitor serum potassium level.
cyclosporine	May increase level of cyclosporine.	• Monitor cyclosporine level.
estrogens	May reduce metabolism of prednisone via increased level of transcortin; may prolong half-life of corticosteroid because of increased protein binding.	• Dosage adjustment may be needed.

insulin oral antidiabetics	Hyperglycemia may occur.	• Monitor serum glucose level. • Monitor patient for signs of hyper- glycemia (fatigue, polyuria, polydipsia, weight loss, abdominal pain, altered mental status, tachycardia, hypotension, glucosuria, ketonuria).
isoniazid salicylates	May increase metabolism of these drugs.	• Dosage adjustment of isoniazid or salicy- lates may be needed.
ulcerogenic drugs	May increase risk of GI ulceration.	• Monitor patient for increased GI com- plaints, abdominal pain, or melena. • Use together cautiously.

primaquine phosphate

aluminum salts magnesium	May decrease GI absorption.	• Separate administration times.
quinacrine	May potentiate toxic effects of primaquine.	• Don't use together.

primidone • Mysoline

acetazolamide succinimides	May decrease level of primidone.	• Monitor serum primidone and phenobar- bital levels. • Separate administration times. • Dosage adjustment or withdrawal of one of these drugs may be needed.
carbamazepine phenytoin	May decrease effects of primidone and in- crease conversion to phenobarbital.	• Monitor patient for clinical effects. • Monitor serum levels to prevent toxicity. • Monitor patient for signs of phenobarbi- tal toxicity, including ataxia, slurred speech, sustained nystagmus, somno- lence, confusion, respiratory depression, pulmonary edema, areflexia, and coma.

(continued)

INTERACTING AGENTS	POSSIBLE EFFECTS	NURSING CONSIDERATIONS
primidone (continued)		
alcohol CNS depressants (such as narcotic analgesics)	May cause excessive depression.	• Avoid use together if possible. • If used together, monitor patient for increased sedation, dizziness, agitation, asthenia, and respiratory depression. • Advise patient to avoid alcohol.
oral contraceptives	Barbiturates may render oral contraceptives ineffective.	• Advise patient to use barrier contraception.
warfarin **oral anticoagulants**	May enhance enzymatic degradation of these drugs.	• Increased doses of anticoagulants may be needed. • Monitor PT and INR.
theophylline	May decrease theophylline level.	• Monitor serum theophylline level. • Dosage adjustment may be needed.
probenecid • Benemid		
aminosalicylic acid dapsone **methotrexate** nitrofurantoin ,	May increase serum levels; may increase risk of toxicity of these drugs.	• Don't use together, if possible. • Nitrofurantoin should not be given concomitantly. • Monitor serum levels or clinical effects if appropriate. • Monitor patient for increased adverse effects of these drugs or toxicity.
bumetanide ethacrynic acid furosemide	May impair natriuretic effects of these drugs.	• Monitor for decreased effect. • Dosage adjustment may be needed.
beta-lactam antibiotics cephalosporins ketamine	May significantly increase or prolong effects of these drugs.	• Probenecid may be used for a therapeutic advantage when given with cephalosporins, penicillins, and other beta-

penicillins sulfonamides thiopental		lactam antibiotics. There is no therapeutic benefit when used with sulfonamides. • Monitor patient for increased adverse effects of these drugs. • Lower dosages of ketamine and thiopental may achieve the desired effect when used with probenecid.
chlorpropamide oral sulfonylureas	May enhance hypoglycemic effects.	• Monitor serum glucose level closely. • Monitor patient for signs of hypoglycemia, including dizziness, diaphoresis, confusion, and tachycardia. • Dosage adjustment may be needed.
alcohol diuretics pyrazinamide	May decrease uric acid levels of probenecid.	• Increased doses of probenecid may be needed. • Advise patient to avoid alcohol.
indomethacin naproxen	May decrease excretion of these drugs.	• Monitor patient for increased adverse effects. • Dosage adjustment may be needed.
ketorolac	May decrease clearance of ketorolac.	• Don't use together.
salicylates	May inhibit uricosuric effect of probenecid only in doses that achieve levels of ≥ 50 mcg/ml; occasional use of low-dose aspirin doesn't interfere.	• Low-dose aspirin may be used in patients taking probenecid.
weak organic acids	May inhibit urinary excretion of these drugs.	• Monitor patient for increased adverse effects.
zidovudine	May increase bioavailability of zidovudine.	• Monitor patient for adverse effects, including cutaneous eruptions accompanied by systemic symptoms (including malaise, myalgia, fever).

INTERACTING AGENTS	POSSIBLE EFFECTS	NURSING CONSIDERATIONS
procainamide hydrochloride • Procanbid, Pronestyl, Pronestyl-SR		
anticholinergics (atropine, diphenhydramine, TCAs)	May cause additive anticholinergic effects.	• Monitor patient for increased anticholinergic effects, such as agitation, confusion, hallucinations, hyperthermia, seizures, urinary retention, pupillary dilatation, dry mucous membranes, pupillary dilation, and constipation.
antihypertensives	May cause additive hypotensive effects (most common with I.V. procainamide).	• Monitor BP.
cholinergics (neostigmine, pyridostigmine, which are used to treat myasthenia gravis)	May negate effects of these drugs.	• Avoid use together, if possible. • If used together, dosages of these drugs may need to be increased.
cimetidine	May impair renal clearance of procainamide and NAPA, with elevated serum drug levels.	• Monitor serum drug levels. • Dosage adjustment may be needed.
neuromuscular blockers (such as decamethonium bromide, gallium triethiodide, metocurine iodide, pancuronium bromide, succinylcholine chloride, tubocurarine chloride)	May potentiate effects of neuromuscular blockers.	• Avoid using together if possible. • If used concomitantly, monitor patient's vital signs, respiratory status, and the return of spontaneous muscle control.
antiarrhythmics	May cause additive or antagonistic cardiac effects and additive toxic effects.	• Monitor drug levels. • Monitor patient for signs of toxicity, such as prolonged QT or QRS intervals, arrhythmias, hypotension, visual disturbances, seizures, ataxia, lethargy, nausea, or vomiting. • Dosage adjustments may be needed.

quinolones	May increase potential to prolong the QT interval.	• Don't use together.
jimsonweed	May cause adverse effect on CV system function.	• Advise patient against concomitant use. • Advise patient to contact health care professional before using any herbs.
licorice	May cause prolonged QT interval; potentially additive.	• Advise patient against concomitant use. • Advise patient to contact health care professional before using any herbs.

prochlorperazine • Compazine, Stemetil†
prochlorperazine edisylate • Compazine
prochlorperazine maleate • Compazine, Compazine Spansule, Stemetil†

antacids containing aluminum and magnesium	May inhibit absorption.	• Separate administration times by at least 2 hr.
antidiarrheals	May increase risk of arrhythmias and conduction defects.	• Use together cautiously. • Monitor vital signs and ECG closely. • Don't use sparfloxacin with prochlorperazine.
antiarrhythmics disopyramide procainamide quinidine quinolones (sparfloxacin)	May cause oversedation, paralytic ileus, visual changes, and severe constipation.	• Use these drugs together only when needed. • Monitor patient closely for adverse effects. • Dosage adjustment or withdrawal of drugs may be needed.

(continued)

INTERACTING AGENTS	POSSIBLE EFFECTS	NURSING CONSIDERATIONS
prochlorperazine *(continued)*		
anticholinergics (such as antidepressants, antihistamines, antiparkinsonians, MAO inhibitors, meperidine, phenothiazines) atropine	May inhibit prochlorperazine metabolism, increasing plasma level and toxicity.	• Dosage adjustment may be needed.
beta blockers	Prochlorperazine may antagonize the therapeutic effect of bromocriptine on prolactin secretion.	• Don't use together, if possible. • Monitor patient for clinical effect. • May need to increase bromocriptine dose.
bromocriptine	May inhibit BP response.	• Monitor BP carefully. • Dosage adjustment or withdrawal of drugs may be needed.
centrally acting antihypertensives (such as clonidine, guanabenz, guanadrel, guanethidine, methyldopa, reserpine)	May cause oversedation, respiratory depression, and hypotension.	• Monitor patient closely for signs of increased CNS depression, including increased sedation, headache, dizziness, ataxia, confusion, agitation, respiratory depression, and hypotension. • Advise patient to avoid alcohol.
alcohol CNS depressants (such as anesthetics [epidural, general, spinal], barbiturates, narcotics, parenteral magnesium sulfate, tranquilizers)	May decrease vasoconstricting effects.	• Monitor patient closely for clinical response.
high-dose dopamine	May decrease effectiveness of levodopa.	• Monitor patient for clinical response to levodopa.
levodopa	May cause severe neurologic toxicity with an encephalitis-like syndrome and a decreased response to prochlorperazine.	• Monitor patient closely. • Dosage reduction or withdrawal of one or both drugs may be needed.

lithium	May increase risk of seizures.	• Monitor patient closely for increased seizures.
metrizamide	May cause hypotension.	• Monitor BP.
nitrates	May enhance renal excretion of prochlorperazine.	• Dosage adjustment may be needed.
phenobarbital	May inhibit metabolism and increase toxicity of phenytoin.	• Monitor serum phenytoin level. • Monitor patient for signs of phenytoin toxicity, including drowsiness, confusion or decreased level of consciousness, nausea, vomiting, nystagmus, ataxia, dysarthria, tremor, slurred speech, hypotension, arrhythmias, and respiratory depression.
phenytoin	May increase risk of agranulocytosis.	• Monitor hematologic studies.
propylthiouracil	May decrease therapeutic response to prochlorperazine.	• Monitor patient for therapeutic effect. • Dosage adjustment may be needed.
caffeine smoking (heavy)	May increase prochlorperazine metabolism.	• Discourage smoking.
sun exposure	May cause photosensitivity reactions.	• Advise patient to use sunblock.

promethazine hydrochloride • Anergan 25, Anergan 50, Histantil†, Phencen-50, Phenergan, Phenergan Fortis, Phenergan Plain, Phenoject-50, V-Gan-25, V-Gan-50

| epinephrine | May cause partial adrenergic blockade and further hypotension. | • Monitor BP. |

(continued)

INTERACTING AGENTS	POSSIBLE EFFECTS	NURSING CONSIDERATIONS
promethazine hydrochloride *(continued)*		
levodopa	May block levodopa's antiparkinsonian action.	• Monitor patient for clinical response to levodopa.
MAO inhibitors	May interfere with detoxification of antihistamines and phenothiazines. May prolong and intensify sedative and anticholinergic effects. May increase risk of extrapyramidal effects.	• Don't use together. • Monitor patient for increased adverse effects.
alcohol antihistamines CNS depressants (anxiolytics, barbiturates, sleeping aids, tranquilizers)	May cause additive CNS depression.	• Monitor patient closely for signs of increased CNS depression, including increased sedation, headache, dizziness, ataxia, confusion, agitation, respiratory depression, and hypotension. • Advise patient to avoid alcohol.
barbituate anesthetics (methohexital, thiopental)	May increase neuromuscular excitation and hypotension.	• Don't give promethazine as a preanesthetic to patients receiving these anesthetics.
quinolones (sparfloxacin)	May increase risk of arrhythmias and conduction defects.	• Don't use together.
sun exposure	May cause photosensitivity reactions.	• Advise patient to use sunblock.
propantheline bromide • Pro-Banthine, Propanthel†		
antacids	May decrease oral absorption of anticholinergics.	• Give propantheline at least 1 hr before antacids.
atenolol	May increase absorption. May enhance atenolol effects.	• Monitor patient for increased effects. • Dosage adjustment may be needed.

digoxin	Slowly dissolving digoxin tablets may yield a higher serum digoxin level.	• Monitor serum digoxin level. • Monitor patients for signs of digoxin toxicity, including fatigue, asthenia, dizziness, arrhythmias, visual disturbances, nausea, vomiting, and diarrhea.
anticholinergics	May cause additive toxicity because of decreased GI motility from anticholinergic effects, resulting in increased digoxin absorption time.	• Monitor patient for increased anticholinergic effects, such as agitation, confusion, hallucinations, hyperthermia, seizures, urinary retention, pupillary dilatation, dry mucous membranes, pupillary dilation, and constipation.
ketoconazole levodopa	May decrease GI absorption of these drugs.	• Separate administration times. • Monitor patient for clinical effect. • Dosage adjustment may be needed.
oral potassium supplements (especially wax-matrix formulations)	May increase potassium-induced GI ulcerations.	• Separate administration times. • Monitor patient for abdominal pain, distension, vomiting, GI bleeding, and melena.

propoxyphene hydrochloride • Darvon
propoxyphene napsylate • Darvocet-N 50, Darvocet-N 100, Darvon-N

antidepressants (such as doxepin)	Propoxyphene may inhibit metabolism of these drugs.	• Monitor patient for increased adverse effects. • Antidepressant dosage may need to be reduced.
carbamazepine	May increase carbamazepine's effects.	• Monitor serum carbamazepine levels. • Monitor patient for toxicity (dizziness, ataxia, respiratory depression, arrhythmias, BP changes, impaired consciousness, restlessness, abnormal reflexes, *(continued)*

INTERACTING AGENTS	POSSIBLE EFFECTS	NURSING CONSIDERATIONS
propoxyphene hydrochloride (continued)		
carbamazepine (continued)		seizures, nausea, vomiting, urinary retention).
cimetidine	May enhance respiratory and CNS depression and cause confusion, disorientation, apnea, or seizures.	• Monitor patient for these effects. • Dosage may need to be adjusted or drug stopped.
drugs highly metabolized in liver (digitoxin, phenytoin, rifampin)	May cause accumulation of either drug. Withdrawal symptoms may result.	• Monitor patient for clinical effect and toxicity. • Dosage may need to be adjusted or drug stopped.
general anesthetics	May cause severe CV depression.	• Monitor vital signs and ECG closely.
opiate antagonist	Patients who become physically dependent on propoxyphene may experience acute withdrawal syndrome when given a single dose.	• Avoid use together, if possible.
CNS depressants (antidepressants, antihistamines, barbiturates, benzodiazepines, general anesthetics, muscle relaxants, narcotic analgesics, phenothiazines, sedative-hypnotics) alcohol	May potentiate adverse effects (respiratory depression, sedation, hypotension).	• Use together cautiously. • Monitor patient closely for increased sedation, dizziness, ataxia, tremor, agitation, respiratory depression, and hypotension. • Reduced doses of propoxyphene are usually needed. • Advise patient to avoid alcohol.
propranolol hydrochloride • Inderal, Inderal LA		
aluminum hydroxide antacids	May decrease GI absorption.	• Separate administration times.
antidiabetics	May prolong hypoglycemia, resulting in al-	• Monitor serum glucose level closely.

insulin	tered dosage requirements in previously stable diabetic patients.	• Monitor patient carefully for signs of hypoglycemia, including dizziness, diaphoresis, confusion, and tachycardia. • Dosage adjustment may be needed.
atropine anticholinergics TCAs	May antagonize propranolol-induced bradycardia.	• Monitor HR.
calcium channel blockers (especially **I.V. verapamil**)	May depress myocardial contractility or AV conduction.	• Use together cautiously. • Monitor vital signs and cardiac function closely. • Dosage adjustments may be needed.
cimetidine	May decrease clearance of propranolol via inhibition of hepatic metabolism.	• Monitor patient for enhanced beta-blocking effects. • Dosage adjustments may be needed.
clonidine	May cause severe hypertension.	• Monitor BP when concomitant therapy starts or stops. • If drug change is warranted, gradually stop the beta blocker first and monitor BP.
epinephrine	May cause severe vasoconstriction followed by bradycardia.	• Don't use together, if possible. • If epinephrine therapy is anticipated, stop propranolol 3 days in advance. • Monitor cardiac function and vital signs closely.
NSAIDs	May antagonize hypotensive effects.	• Monitor BP.

(continued)

Interacting agents in **bold type** indicate severe, well-documented interactions.   †Canadian

INTERACTING AGENTS	POSSIBLE EFFECTS	NURSING CONSIDERATIONS
propranolol hydrochloride *(continued)*		
phenytoin rifampin	May accelerate clearance of propranolol.	• Monitor patient for clinical effect. • Dosage adjustments may be needed.
sympathomimetics (such as isoproterenol, MAO inhibitors)	May antagonize beta-adrenergic stimulating effects.	• Monitor patient for clinical effects.
tubocurarine and related compounds	High doses of propranolol may potentiate neuromuscular blocking effect.	• Monitor patient closely, especially for increased respiratory depression.

antihypertensives (especially cate-
  cholamine-depleting drugs, such as
  reserpine)
	May potentiate antihypertensive effects.	• Monitor BP.

betel palm	May reduce temperature-elevating effects and enhance CNS effects.	• Advise patient to avoid use together. • Advise patient to consult health care provider before taking herbal preparations.
alcohol	May slow rate of absorption.	• Advise patient to avoid alcohol.
pseudoephedrine sulfate • Cenafed, Decofed, Efidac/24, Genaphed, Novafed, PediaCare Infants' Decongestant Drops, Pseudogest, Sudafed, Triaminic AM		
beta blockers	May increase pressor effects of pseudoephedrine.	• Monitor BP.
methyldopa reserpine	May reduce antihypertensive effects.	• Monitor BP.
MAO inhibitors TCAs	May potentiate pressor effects of pseudoephedrine.	• Don't use together. • Allow at least 14 days after stopping MAO inhibitor before using pseudoephedrine.

		• If using with a TCA, monitor patient for arrhythmias and hypertension.
		• Dosage adjustment may be needed.
sympathomimetics	May cause additive effects.	• Avoid use together, if possible.
		• Monitor patient for toxicity if used together.

quetiapine fumarate • Seroquel

antihypertensives	May potentiate the hypotensive effect of both drugs.	• Monitor BP.
cimetidine phenytoin thioridazine	May increase the mean oral clearance of quetiapine.	• Monitor patient for clinical effect.
		• Quetiapine dose may need adjustment.
CNS depressants	May increase CNS effects.	• Monitor patient closely for increased CNS depressant effects (sedation, dizziness, ataxia, tremor, agitation, respiratory depression).
dopamine agonists levodopa	Quetiapine may antagonize the effect of these drugs.	• Monitor patient closely for clinical effects.
erythromycin fluconazole itraconazole ketoconazole	May decrease quetiapine clearance.	• Monitor patient for signs of toxicity, including increased drowsiness, sedation, tachycardia, hypotension, electrolyte disturbances, and arrhythmias.
lorazepam	May reduce clearance.	• Monitor patient closely for increased adverse effects, such as sedation, dizziness,

(continued)

INTERACTING AGENTS	POSSIBLE EFFECTS	NURSING CONSIDERATIONS
quetiapine fumarate *(continued)*		
lorazepam *(continued)*		ataxia, tremor, agitation, or respiratory depression. • Lorazepam dose may need to be adjusted.
alcohol	May potentiate cognitive and motor effects.	• Advise patient to avoid alcohol.
quinapril hydrochloride • Accupril		
antihypertensives diuretics	May increase risk of excessive hypotension.	• May need to stop the diuretic or lower quinapril dose.
lithium	May increase risk of hyperkalemia.	• Monitor serum lithium level. • Monitor patient for signs of toxicity, including sedation, confusion, tremors, muscle stiffness, increased deep tendon reflexes, visual changes, and nystagmus.
potassium supplements potassium-containing salt substitutes potassium-sparing diuretics	May increase serum lithium level and potentiate lithium toxicity.	• Monitor renal function test results and potassium level. • Monitor patient for signs of hyperkalemia, including mental confusion, neuromuscular excitability, weakness, paresthesia, ascending flaccid paralysis, peaked T waves, depressed ST segment, absence of P wave, prolonged QT interval, and widened QRS complex. • Advise patient to avoid salt substitutes containing potassium.
tetracycline	May significantly impair absorption of tetracycline, potentially from the magnesium content in the quinapril.	• Don't use together. • If unavoidable, monitor patient for clinical effect.

amiloride	May reverse quinidine's antiarrhythmic effects.	• Don't use together.
antacids sodium bicarbonate thiazide diuretics	May decrease quinidine elimination when urine pH increases, requiring close monitoring of therapy.	• Monitor serum quinidine level. • Monitor patient for increased adverse effects, including vertigo, seizures, cardiac arrhythmias, hypotension, respiratory distress, and hematologic abnormalities.
anticholinergics	May lead to additive anticholinergic effects.	• Use together cautiously. • Monitor patient for increased adverse effects.
anticonvulsants (such as phenobarbital and phenytoin)	May increase the rate of quinidine metabolism, leading to a decreased quinidine level.	• Monitor serum quinidine level. • Monitor patient for clinical effect.
cholinergics	May fail to terminate paroxysmal supraventricular tachycardia. Anticholinergic effects of quinidine may negate the effects of these drugs when used to treat myasthenia gravis. Quinidine antagonizes the effects of cholinergic drugs on the vagus nerve.	• Avoid quinidine use in myasthenia gravis patients, if possible. • If used together, anticholinesterase drugs may need to be increased.
coumarin	May potentiate anticoagulant effect of coumarin, leading to hypoprothrombinemic hemorrhage.	• Monitor PT and INR. • Monitor patient for increased bleeding tendencies.
digoxin	May cause increased (possibly toxic) serum digoxin level.	• When quinidine therapy starts, digoxin dosage may need to be reduced by 50%. • Monitor serum digoxin level.

(continued)

INTERACTING AGENTS	POSSIBLE EFFECTS	NURSING CONSIDERATIONS
quinidine gluconatem (continued)		
hypotensives	May cause additive hypotensive effects, mainly when given I.V.	• Monitor BP closely.
neuromuscular blockers (such as metocurine iodide, pancuronium bromide, succinylcholine chloride, tubocurarine chloride)	May potentiate anticholinergic effects.	• Don't use quinidine immediately after using these drugs. • If unavoidable, respiratory support may be needed.
antiarrhythmics (such as **amiodarone**, lidocaine, phenytoin, procainamide, propranolol)	May cause additive or antagonistic cardiac effects and additive toxic effects.	• Monitor serum quinidine level closely. • Dosage adjustment may be needed. • Use with caution.
phenothiazines reserpine	May cause additive cardiac-depressant effects.	• Monitor ECG and vital signs closely.
quinolones (sparfloxacin)	May increase risk of arrhythmias and conduction defects.	• Don't use together.
rifampin	May increase quinidine metabolism and decrease serum quinidine level.	• Monitor serum quinidine level. • Dosage adjustment may be needed when rifampin therapy starts or stops.
nifedipine	May decrease quinidine level.	• Monitor serum quinidine levels.
verapamil	May result in significant hypotension in patients with hypertrophic cardiomyopathy. Ventricular tachycardia, bradycardia, and AV block may also occur.	• Don't use together, if possible. • If used together, monitor patient carefully.
jimsonweed	May adversely affect CV function.	• Advise patient to avoid use. • Advise patient to consult health care provider before taking herbal preparations.

licorice	May prolong the QT interval and cause potentially additive effects.	• Advise patient to avoid use. • Advise patient to consult health care provider before taking herbal preparations.
grapefruit juice	May delay absorption of quinidine.	• Drug shouldn't be taken with grapefruit juice.

raloxifene hydrochloride • Evista

cholestyramine	May cause a significant reduction in absorption of raloxifene.	• Don't give together.
highly protein-bound drugs (such as clofibrate, diazepam, diazoxide, ibuprofen, indomethacin, naproxen)	May interfere with binding sites.	• Use together cautiously. • Monitor patient for clinical effects.
warfarin	May decrease PT.	• Monitor PT and INR.

ramipril • Altace

diuretics	May increase risk of excessive hypotension.	• Dose reduction of ramipril or withdrawal of diuretic may be needed.
lithium	May increase serum lithium level and potentiate lithium toxicity.	• Monitor serum lithium level. • Monitor patient for signs of toxicity, including sedation, confusion, tremors, muscle stiffness, increased deep tendon reflexes, visual changes, and nystagmus.
potassium supplements potassium-containing salt substitutes potassium-sparing diuretics	May increase risk of hyperkalemia.	• Monitor renal function test results and serum potassium level. • Signs of hyperkalemia include confusion, neuromuscular excitability, weakness, paresthesia, and ECG changes. • Advise patient to avoid salt substitutes containing potassium.
sun exposure	May cause photosensitivity reaction.	• Advise patient to use sunblock.

Interacting agents in **bold type** indicate severe, well-documented interactions.   †Canadian

INTERACTING AGENTS	POSSIBLE EFFECTS	NURSING CONSIDERATIONS
ranitidine • Zantac, Zantac 75, Zantac EFFERdose, Zantac GELdose		
antacids	May decrease ranitidine absorption.	• Give drugs at least 1 hr apart. • Monitor closely.
diazepam	May decrease diazepam absorption.	• Monitor patient for clinical effects. • Separate administration times.
glipizide	May increase hypoglycemic effect.	• Dosage adjustment of glipizide may be needed. • Observe patient for signs of excessive hypoglycemia (dizziness, diaphoresis, confusion, tachycardia).
procainamide	May decrease renal clearance of procainamide.	• Monitor patient closely for increased adverse effects and toxicity.
warfarin	May interfere with clearance of warfarin.	• Monitor PT and INR.
repaglinide • Prandin		
barbiturates carbamazepine rifampin troglitazone	May increase repaglinide metabolism.	• Monitor serum glucose level. • Monitor patient for signs of hyperglycemia or hypoglycemia. • Dosage adjustment may be needed.
beta blockers chloramphenicol coumarin highly protein-bound drugs MAO inhibitors NSAIDs probenecid salicylates sulfonamides	May potentiate the hypoglycemic action of repaglinide.	• Monitor serum glucose level closely. • Monitor patient carefully for signs of hypoglycemia, including dizziness, headache, diaphoresis, confusion, and tachycardia. • Dosage adjustment may be needed.

calcium channel blockers corticosteroids estrogens isoniazid nicotinic acid oral contraceptives phenothiazines phenytoin sympathomimetics thiazides and other diuretics thyroid hormones	May cause hyperglycemia.	• Monitor serum glucose level. • Monitor patient for signs of hyper- glycemia (fatigue, polyuria, polydipsia, weight loss, abdominal pain, altered mental status, dehydration, electrolyte disturbances, tachycardia, hypotension, glucosuria, ketonuria). • Dosage adjustment may be needed.
erythromycin ketoconazole miconazole similar inhibitors of the P-450 cytochrome system 3A4	May inhibit repaglinide metabolism.	• Monitor serum glucose level. • Monitor patient for adequate blood glu- cose control and for signs of hypo- glycemia.

rifampin • Rifadin, Rimactane

| anticoagulants
barbiturates
beta blockers
cardiac glycoside derivatives
chloramphenicol
clofibrate
corticosteroids
cyclosporine
dapsone
disopyramide
estrogens
methadone
oral contraceptives | May decrease effectiveness of these drugs. | • Don't use corticosteroids with rifampin.
If used together, corticosteroid dose may
need to be doubled.
• Monitor patient closely for expected clin-
ical effects of these drugs.
• Monitor PT and INR.
• Dosage adjustments may be needed
when rifampin is added or withdrawn
from drug regimen.
• Monitor patient for any toxic effects of
these drugs when rifampin is stopped.
• Rifampin inactivates oral contraceptives
and may alter menstrual patterns. |

(continued)

Interacting agents in **bold type** indicate severe, well-documented interactions.   †Canadian

INTERACTING AGENTS	POSSIBLE EFFECTS	NURSING CONSIDERATIONS
rifampin *(continued)*		
oral sulfonylureas phenytoin quinidine tocainide verapamil		• Advise oral contraceptive users to use barrier contraception.
alcohol **isoniazid**	May increase hazard of hepatotoxicity.	• Monitor liver function test results. • Monitor patient for signs of hepatotoxicity (jaundice, fever, abdominal pain, clay-colored stools, tea-colored urine). • Advise patient to avoid alcohol.
para-aminosalicylate	May decrease oral absorption of rifampin, lowering serum level.	• Give drugs 8 to 12 hr apart.
rifapentine • Priftin		
antiarrhythmics (such as disopyramide, mexiletine, quinidine, tocainide) antibiotics (such as chloramphenicol, clarithromycin, dapsone, doxycycline, fluoroquinolones) anticonvulsants (such as phenytoin) antifungals (such as fluconazole, itraconazole, ketoconazole) barbiturates benzodiazepines (such as diazepam) beta blockers calcium channel blockers (such as diltiazem, nifedipine, verapamil) cardiac glycosides	Rifapentine decreases the activity of these drugs and increases their hepatic metabolism.	• Avoid using corticosteroids with rifapentine. If used together, corticosteroid dose may need to be doubled. • Rifapentine should be used very cautiously or not at all in patients taking protease inhibitors. • Monitor patient closely for expected clinical effects of any of these drugs. • Monitor serum levels of appropriate drugs. • Monitor PT and INR. • Dosage adjustments may be needed when rifapentine is added or withdrawn from drug regimen.

corticosteroids
clofibrate
haloperidol
HIV protease inhibitors (such as indinavir,
    nelfinavir, ritonavir, saquinavir)
immunosuppressants (such as cyclo-
    sporine and tacrolimus)
levothyroxine
narcotic analgesics (such as methadone)
oral anticoagulants (such as warfarin)
oral hypoglycemics (such as sulfony-
    lureas)
oral or other systemic hormonal contra-
    ceptives
progestins
quinine
reverse transcriptase inhibitors (such as
    delavirdine and zidovudine)
sildenafil
theophylline
TCAs (such as amitriptyline and nortripty-
    line)

- Patient should be monitored for any
  toxic effects of these drugs when
  rifapentine is stopped.
- Rifapentine inactivates oral contracep-
  tives and may alter menstrual patterns.
- Advise oral contraceptive users to use
  barrier contraception.

risperidone • Risperdal

antihypertensives	May enhance the effects of certain antihy-pertensives.	• Monitor BP closely.
carbamazepine	May increase risperidone clearance, de-creasing the effectiveness of risperi-done.	• Monitor patient closely for clinical effects when starting or stopping carba-mazepine. • Dosage adjustments may be needed.

(continued)

INTERACTING AGENTS	POSSIBLE EFFECTS	NURSING CONSIDERATIONS
risperidone *(continued)*		
clozapine	May decrease risperidone clearance, increasing the risk of toxicity.	• Monitor patient closely for signs of toxicity, including drowsiness, sedation, tachycardia, hypotension, extrapyramidal symptoms, hyponatremia, hypokalemia, prolonged QT interval and widened QRS complex, and seizures.
alcohol CNS depressants	May cause additive CNS depression.	• Use together cautiously. • Monitor patient closely for increased CNS depressant effects, such as sedation, dizziness, ataxia, tremor, agitation, and respiratory depression.
dopamine agonists levodopa	Risperidone may antagonize the effects of these drugs.	• Don't use together, if possible. • If drugs are used together, monitor patient for clinical effects.
sun exposure	May cause photosensitivity reactions.	• Advise patient to use sunblock.
ritonavir • Norvir		
drugs that increase CYP3A activity (such as carbamazepine, dexamethasone, phenobarbital, phenytoin, rifabutin, rifampin)	May increase ritonavir clearance, resulting in decreased ritonavir plasma level.	• Don't give ritonavir with rifampin. • Monitor patient for clinical effect if used with other drugs.
alprazolam clorazepate diazepam estazolam flurazepam midazolam	May increase potential for extreme sedation and respiratory depression from these drugs.	• Don't give ritonavir with midazolam or triazolam. • Don't use with other drugs, if possible. • If used together, monitor patient closely for increased sedation, dizziness, ataxia, tremor, agitation, and respiratory de-

triazolam zolpidem		pression. • Dosage reduction of these drugs may be needed.
alprazolam methadone	May decrease levels of these drugs.	• Monitor patient for clinical effects. • Dosage adjustment may be needed.
amiodarone bepridil bupropion carbamazepine cisapride clonazepam clozapine encainide ergot alkaloids ethosuximide flecainide meperidine pimozide piroxicam propafenone propoxyphene quinidine rifabutin	May significantly increase plasma levels of these drugs, increasing the patient's risk of arrhythmias, hematologic abnormalities, seizures, or other potentially serious adverse effects.	• Don't use amiodarone, bepridil, clozapine, encainide, flecainide, propafenone, quinidine, ergot alkaloids, cisapride, meperidine, pimozide, or rifabutin with ritonavir. • Dosages of other drugs may need to be reduced to avoid increased adverse reactions. • If used together, monitor patient closely.
clarithromycin	May reduce creatinine clearance.	• Patients with creatinine clearance of 30 to 60 ml/min may need clarithromycin dose reduced by 50%. Those with creatinine clearance below 30 ml/min may need a 75% reduction.

(continued)

Interacting agents in **bold type** indicate severe, well-documented interactions.   †Canadian

INTERACTING AGENTS	POSSIBLE EFFECTS	NURSING CONSIDERATIONS
ritonavir *(continued)*		
desipramine	May increase serum level of desipramine.	• Monitor desipramine level. • Dosage adjustment may be needed.
disopyramide mexiletine nefazodone fluoxetine beta blockers	Cardiac and neurologic events may occur.	• Dosage reduction of these drugs may be needed when given with ritonavir.
disulfiram or other drugs that produce disulfiram-like reactions (such as metronidazole)	Ritonavir formulations contain alcohol that can produce reactions; may increase risk of disulfiram-like reactions.	• Monitor patient.
glucuronosyltransferases (including oral anticoagulants or immunosuppressants)	May cause loss of therapeutic effects from directly glucuronidated drugs. Immunosuppressants such as cyclosporine and tacrolimus may have significantly increased plasma levels.	• Monitor drug levels. • Monitor patient for drug effects. • A dosage change of these drugs may be needed. A dosage reduction greater than 50% may be required for those drugs extensively metabolized by CYP3A4.
HMG-CoA reductase inhibitors (such as atorvastatin, lovastatin, simvastatin)	May increase risk of myopathy, including rhabdomyolysis.	• If these drugs must be used together, monitor patient for signs of myopathy and rhabdomyolysis (increased serum creatinine kinase level, muscle aches, weakness).
ketoconazole	May increase level of ritonavir.	• Monitor patient for adverse effects.
ketoconazole sildenafil	May increase levels of these drugs.	• Avoid using more than 200 mg/day of ketoconazole. • Patients should not receive more than a 25-mg single dose of sildenafil in a 48-hr period.

oral contraceptives	May decrease serum level of the contraceptive.	• May require a dosage increase of the oral contraceptive or alternate contraceptive measures.
divalproex lamotrigine phenytoin	May decrease serum levels of these drugs.	• Monitor patient for loss of seizure control. • Monitor serum level of ritonavir.
theophylline	May decrease serum theophylline level.	• Monitor serum theophylline level. • Increased dosage may be needed.
St. John's wort	May substantially reduce blood level of the drug and cause loss of therapeutic effects.	• Warn against concomitant use. • If drug levels are adjusted for a patient already taking St. John's wort, stopping the herb could cause blood levels to rise to toxic levels. • Advise patient to contact health care professional before using any herbal preparations.
food	May increase absorption.	• Drug should be taken with food.
smoking	May decrease serum level of ritonavir.	• Discourage smoking.
rofecoxib • Vioxx		
ACE inhibitors	May decrease antihypertensive effects of ACE inhibitor.	• Monitor patient for clinical effect. • Monitor BP.
alcohol use (long-term) aspirin smoking	May increase rate of GI ulceration.	• Monitor patient for increased GI complaints, abdominal pain, melena, and GI bleeding.

(continued)

INTERACTING AGENTS	POSSIBLE EFFECTS	NURSING CONSIDERATIONS
rofecoxib *(continued)*		
alcohol use (long-term), aspirin, smoking (continued)		• Discourage alcohol use and smoking. • Don't use together.
furosemide thiazide diuretics	May decrease effectiveness of these drugs; diuretics may increase nephrotoxicity.	• Monitor BP and renal function test results.
lithium methotrexate	May increase plasma lithium level and decrease lithium clearance; may increase plasma methotrexate level.	• For lithium, monitor patient for signs of toxicity, including sedation, confusion, tremors, muscle stiffness, increased deep tendon reflexes, visual changes, and nystagmus. • For methotrexate, monitor patient for myelosuppression, anemia, nausea, vomiting, diarrhea, dermatitis, alopecia, melena, and fatigue. • Monitor serum levels of these drugs.
rifampin	May decrease rofecoxib level by about 50%.	• Start therapy with a higher dosage of rofecoxib.
warfarin	May increase effects of warfarin.	• Monitor PT and INR frequently in the first few days after therapy with rofecoxib is started or changed.
ropinirole hydrochloride • Requip		
alcohol CNS depressants (including antipsychotics and benzodiazepines)	May increase CNS effects.	• Monitor patient closely for increased sedation, dizziness, ataxia, tremor, agitation, and respiratory depression. • Advise patient to avoid alcohol.
dopamine antagonists (including butyrophenones, metoclopramide, pheno-	May decrease effectiveness of ropinirole.	• Don't use together, if possible. • If used together, monitor patient for clin-

thiazines, thioxanthenes)		ical effect.
estrogens	May reduce clearance of ropinirole.	• Dosage adjustment of ropinirole may be needed.
inhibitors or substrates of cytochrome P-450 CYP1A2 (such as ciprofloxacin, fluvoxamine, mexiletine, norfloxacin)	May alter clearance of ropinirole.	• Dosage adjustment of ropinirole may be needed.
smoking	May increase clearance of ropinirole.	• Discourage smoking.

scopolamine hydrobromide • Isopto Hyoscine, Scopace, Transderm-Scop

ketoconazole levodopa	May decrease GI absorption of these drugs.	• Separate administration times by 2 to 3 hr.
alcohol CNS depressants (including sedative-hypnotics and tranquilizers)	May increase CNS depression.	• Use together cautiously. • Monitor patient for increased sedation, headache, dizziness, agitation, asthenia, and respiratory depression. • Advise patient to avoid alcohol.
digoxin	May cause a higher serum digoxin level.	• Monitor serum digoxin level. • Monitor patient for signs of digoxin toxicity, including fatigue, asthenia, dizziness, arrhythmias, visual disturbances, nausea, vomiting, and diarrhea.
anticholinergics (such as belladonna alkaloids, antihistamines, TCAs, muscle relaxants)	May cause additive toxicity.	• Avoid use together, if possible. • When drugs are used together, monitor patients for signs of toxicity, including mental status changes, hallucinations, xerostomia, visual disturbances, dilated pupils, tachycardia, ECG changes, hyperthermia, hypertension, increased respiratory rate, urinary retention, and constipation.

(continued)

INTERACTING AGENTS	POSSIBLE EFFECTS	NURSING CONSIDERATIONS
scopolamine hydrobromide *(continued)*		
anticholinergics *(continued)*		• Dosage adjustments may be needed to avoid toxicity.
oral potassium supplements, especially wax-matrix formulations	May increase potassium-induced GI ulcerations.	• Use together cautiously. • Monitor patient for increased GI complaints, abdominal pain, and melena.
phenothiazines	May decrease effects of phenothiazines.	• Monitor patient for clinical effects. • Phenothiazine dosage adjustment may be needed.
jaborandi tree pill-bearing spurge	May decrease effects.	• Advise patient against concomitant use. • Advise patient to contact health care professional before using any herbal preparations.
squaw vine	Tannic acid in squaw vine may decrease metabolic breakdown of scopolamine.	• Advise patient against concomitant use. • Advise patient to contact health care professional before using any herbal preparations.
sun exposure	With ophthalmic form, photophobia may occur.	• Advise patient to use sunblock.
selegiline hydrochloride (L-deprenyl hydrochloride) • Eldepryl, Carbex		
adrenergics	May increase the vasopressor response.	• Monitor BP closely. • Monitor patient for symptoms of hypertensive crisis, such as headache, dizziness, palpitations, nausea, headache, and chest tightness.
meperidine	Fatal interactions may occur.	• Don't use together.

fluoxetine SSRIs (including citalopram, fluvoxamine, nefazodone, paroxetine, sertraline, venlafaxine)	May result in serotonin syndrome (altered mental status; increased muscle tone, weakness, twitching; hyperthermia; delirium; coma; death).	• Avoid use together. • Allow 5 wk between stopping fluoxetine therapy and starting selegiline therapy. • Allow 2 wk or longer between stopping SSRI therapy and starting selegiline therapy.
ginseng	May cause headache, tremors, and mania.	• Advise patient against using together. • Advise patient to contact health care professional before using any herbal preparations.
cacao	May cause potential vasopressor effects.	• Advise patient against using together. • Advise patient to contact health care professional before using any herbal preparations.
foods high in tyramine	May cause possible hypertensive crisis.	• Advise patient to avoid using together. • If they are taken together, monitor BP. • Monitor patient for symptoms of hypertensive crisis, including headache, dizziness, palpitations, nausea, headache, and chest tightness.
alcohol	Excessive depressant effect is possible.	• Advise patient to avoid alcohol.
sertraline hydrochloride • Zoloft		
cimetidine	May increase sertraline bioavailability, peak plasma level, and half-life.	• Monitor patient closely for increased adverse effects. • Dosage adjustments of sertraline may be needed.
diazepam tolbutamide	May decrease clearance of these drugs by sertraline.	• For diazepam, monitor patient for increased CNS-depressant effects (seda- *(continued)*

INTERACTING AGENTS	POSSIBLE EFFECTS	NURSING CONSIDERATIONS
sertraline hydrochloride *(continued)*		
diazepam, tolbutamide *(continued)*		tion, dizziness, ataxia, tremor, agitation, respiratory depression). • For tolbutamide, monitor patient for signs of excessive hypoglycemia (dizziness, diaphoresis, confusion, tachycardia).
MAO inhibitors sibutramine sumatriptan sympathomimetics	May increase risk of serotonin syndrome (altered mental status; increased muscle tone, weakness, twitching; hyperthermia, delirium, coma, death).	• Drug must not be given within 14 days of an MAO inhibitor. • Don't use with sympathomimetics, sibutramine, or sumatriptan, if possible. • If used together, monitor patient for increased CNS effects.
highly protein-bound drugs warfarin	May cause increased plasma level of sertraline or other highly bound drug.	• Monitor for increased adverse effects of these drugs. • Monitor PT and INR, if applicable.
St. John's wort	May increase serotonin levels, leading to serotonin syndrome (altered mental status; increased muscle tone, weakness, twitching; hyperthermia; delirium; coma; death).	• Warn patient against using together. • Inform patient that a sufficient "washout" period should occur before switching from an SSRI to St. John's wort.
sevelamer hydrochloride • Renagel		
antiarrhythmics anticonvulsants oral medications	May increase potential for decreased bioavailability of drug and decrease therapeutic effects.	• Give other drugs at least 1 hr before or 3 hr after sevelamer.
sibutramine hydrochloride monohydrate • Meridia		
alcohol CNS depressants	May enhance CNS depression.	• Use together cautiously. • Monitor patient for increased sedation,

		headache, dizziness, agitation, asthenia, and respiratory depression.
		• Advise patient to avoid alcohol.
dextromethorphan dihydroergotamine fentanyl fluoxetine fluvoxamine lithium MAO inhibitors meperidine paroxetine pentazocine sertraline sumatriptan tryptophan venlafaxine	May cause hyperthermia, tachycardia, and loss of consciousness.	• Don't use together. • If concomitant use is unavoidable, monitor patient closely for adverse effects. • Don't use sibutramine during or within 2 wk of MAO inhibitor therapy.
inhibitors of cytochrome P-450 3A4 metabolism (such as erythromycin and ketoconazole)	May decrease sibutramine metabolism.	• Monitor patient for increased adverse effects. • Dose of sibutramine may need to be reduced.
ephedrine pseudoephedrine	May increase BP or HR.	• Monitor vital signs and ECG closely.
sildenafil citrate • Viagra		
inhibitors of cytochrome P-450 isoforms 3A4 (such as cimetidine, erythromycin, itraconazole, ketoconazole, protease inhibitors)	May reduce the clearance of sildenafil.	• Use sildenafil with extreme caution in patients taking these drugs. • A reduced dosage of 25 mg in a 48-hr period is recommended.

(continued)

INTERACTING AGENTS	POSSIBLE EFFECTS	NURSING CONSIDERATIONS
sildenafil citrate *(continued)*		
nitrates	May enhance the hypotensive effects of nitrates.	• Don't use together. • Obtain a careful health history of nitrate use before sildenafil therapy.
rifampin	May reduce sildenafil plasma level.	• Monitor sildenafil clinical effects. • Dosage adjustments may be needed.
high-fat meals	May delay absorption of drug and onset of action by 1 hr.	• Advise patient to separate administration time from meals.
simethicone • Gas-X, Mylicon, Phazyme		
alginic acid	May decrease effectiveness of alginic acid.	• Monitor patient for clinical effect.
simvastatin • Zocor		
cimetidine ketoconazole spironolactone	May increase risk of endocrine dysfunction and diminish the levels or activity of steroid hormones.	• Take complete drug history of patient who develops endocrine dysfunction. • No intervention appears needed.
digoxin	Simvastatin may slightly elevate levels.	• Closely monitor serum digoxin level when simvastatin therapy starts.
erythromycin fibric acid derivatives (clofibrate, gemfibrozil) high doses of niacin ($\geq$ 1 g nicotinic acid daily) immunosuppressants (such as cyclosporine) verapamil	May increase risk of rhabdomyolysis.	• Don't use together, if possible. • If unavoidable, monitor patient for signs of myopathy and rhabdomyolysis (increased serum creatinine kinase level, muscle aches, weakness). • Limit daily dose of simvastatin to 10 mg if patient must take cyclosporine.
alcohol hepatotoxic drugs	May increase risk of hepatotoxicity.	• Monitor liver function test results. • Monitor patient for signs of hepatotoxici-

		ty (jaundice, fever, abdominal pain, clay-colored stools, tea-colored urine). • Advise patient to avoid alcohol.
grapefruit juice	May increase simvastatin serum levels and increase adverse effects such as rhabdomyolysis.	• Don't give simvastatin with grapefruit juice.
warfarin	Simvastatin may slightly enhance the anticoagulant effect.	• Monitor PT at the start of therapy and during dose adjustment.

sirolimus • Rapamune

aminoglycosides amphotericin nephrotoxic drugs	May increase risk of nephrotoxicity.	• Avoid using together, if possible. • If used concomitantly, monitor renal function test results.
bromocriptine cimetidine cisapride clarithromycin clotrimazole CYP3A4 inhibitors danazol erythromycin fluconazole grapefruit juice indinavir itraconazole metoclopramide nicardipine ritonavir verapamil	May decrease sirolimus metabolism, increasing sirolimus level.	• Monitor sirolimus level. • Monitor patient for increased adverse effects, including thrombocytopenia, anemia, electrolyte and lipid abnormalities, arrhythmias, hypertension, nausea, vomiting, and diarrhea. • Drug shouldn't be taken with or mixed in grapefruit juice.

(continued)

INTERACTING AGENTS	POSSIBLE EFFECTS	NURSING CONSIDERATIONS
sirolimus (continued)		
carbamazepine CYP3A4 inducers phenobarbital phenytoin rifabutin rifapentine	May increase sirolimus metabolism, decreasing sirolimus blood level.	• Monitor sirolimus levels. • Monitor the patient closely for clinical effect.
cyclosporine (oral solution and capsules)	May increase sirolimus level.	• Give sirolimus 4 hr after cyclosporine. • After long-term administration, sirolimus may reduce cyclosporine clearance, leading to need for reduction in cyclosporine dose.
diltiazem	May increase sirolimus level.	• Monitor patient for increased adverse effects. • Dosage reduction of sirolimus may be needed.
ketoconazole	May increase rate and extent of sirolimus absorption.	• Don't use together.
live virus vaccines (BCG, measles, mumps, oral polio, rubella, TY21a typhoid, varicella, yellow fever)	May reduce effectiveness of vaccines.	• Avoid administering vaccines during therapy.
rifampin	May significantly decrease sirolimus level.	• Avoid using together.
somatropin • Genotropin, Humatrope, Nutropin		
glucocorticoids	May inhibit the effects of growth hormone.	• Monitor patient for clinical effect. • Dosage adjustments may be needed, especially in pediatric patients.

drugs metabolized by CYP450 liver enzymes (such as corticosteroids, sex steroids, anticonvulsants, cyclosporine)	May alter clearance of these drugs.	• Monitor patient for clinical effects and toxicity. • Monitor serum levels. • Monitor patient for clinical effects.

sotalol • Betapace

antacids	May decrease effects of sotalol; may decrease absorption when given with food.	• Advise patient to take 2 hr apart. • Give drug on an empty stomach.
antiarrhythmics	May cause additive effects.	• Monitor patient's ECG and vital signs.
calcium channel antagonists	May enhance myocardial depression.	• Don't use together, if possible. • If unavoidable, monitor cardiac function. • Dosage adjustments may be needed.
catecholamine-depleting drugs (such as guanethidine and reserpine)	May enhance the hypotensive effects of sotalol.	• Monitor BP and HR.
clonidine	Sotalol may enhance the rebound hypertensive effect seen after withdrawal of clonidine.	• Discontinue sotalol several days before withdrawing clonidine.
insulin oral antidiabetics	Hyperglycemia may occur. Symptoms of hypoglycemia may be masked.	• Monitor serum glucose level closely. • Monitor patient for signs of hyperglycemia, including fatigue, polyuria, polydipsia, weight loss, abdominal pain, altered mental status, tachycardia, hypotension, glucosuria, and ketonuria. • Monitor patient carefully for signs of hypoglycemia, including dizziness, diaphoresis, confusion, and tachycardia. • Dosage adjustment may be needed.
NSAIDs	May antagonize hypotensive effects.	• Monitor BP.
quinolones	May increase risk of arrhythmias and conduction defects.	• Don't use sparfloxacin with sotalol.

Interacting agents in **bold type** indicate severe, well-documented interactions.   †Canadian

INTERACTING AGENTS	POSSIBLE EFFECTS	NURSING CONSIDERATIONS
sparfloxacin • Zagam		
antacids containing aluminum or magnesium, iron salts, zinc, or sucralfate	May interfere with GI absorption of sparfloxacin.	• Give at least 4 hr apart.
drugs that prolong the QTc interval (including amiodarone, bepridil, disopyramide, class Ia antiarrhythmics [procainamide, quinidine], class III antiarrhythmics [sotalol]; bepridil, erythromycin, pentamidine, TCAs, and some antipsychotics, including phenothiazines)	May cause torsades de pointes.	• Sparfloxacin is contraindicated for patients taking any drugs that may prolong the QTc interval. • Another quinolone antibiotic that does not prolong the QTc interval or is not metabolized by the CYP3A4 isoenzyme may be considered. • Monitor ECG.
sun exposure	May cause photosensitivity reactions.	• Advise patient to use sunblock.
streptokinase • Streptase		
aminocaproic acid	May inhibit streptokinase-induced activation of plasminogen.	• Don't use together unless using for clinically emergent situation.
anticoagulants	May cause hemorrhage.	• Monitor PTT, PT, aPTT, and INR. • Monitor patient for increased bleeding tendencies (bruising, petechiae, bleeding gums, epistaxis, prolonged bleeding after injury, melena, GI bleeding, hematuria, and hematemesis). • Effects of oral anticoagulants may need to be reversed before beginning streptokinase therapy.
dong quai feverfew garlic ginger	May increase risk of bleeding.	• Discourage use together. • Advise patient to contact health care professional before using any herbs.

horse chestnut
red clover

aspirin drugs affecting platelet activity indomethacin phenylbutazone	May increase risk of bleeding.	• Monitor patient for clinical effects. • Monitor patient for increased bleeding tendencies (bruising, petechiae, bleeding gums, epistaxis, prolonged bleeding after injury, melena, GI bleeding, hematuria, and hematemesis).

streptozocin • Zanosar

doxorubicin	May prolong elimination half-life of doxorubicin.	• Monitor patient for increased adverse effects. • Reduced dose of doxorubicin is needed.
nephrotoxic drugs	May potentiate nephrotoxicity caused by streptozocin.	• Don't use together.
phenytoin	May decrease effects of streptozocin on the pancreas.	• Don't use together, if possible.

sucralfate • Carafate

antacids	May decrease binding of drug to gastroduodenal mucosa, impairing effectiveness.	• Separate dosing of sucralfate and antacids by 30 min.
anticoagulants cimetidine digoxin phenytoin quinidine quinolones ranitidine tetracycline theophylline fat-soluble vitamins A, D, E, and K	Sucralfate may decrease absorption of these drugs.	• Separate administration times by at least 2 hr. For quinolones, separate administration times by at least 6 hr. • Monitor patient for clinical effects of these drugs. • Monitor serum levels of these drugs if applicable. • May need to discontinue sucralfate.

INTERACTING AGENTS	POSSIBLE EFFECTS	NURSING CONSIDERATIONS
sulfamethoxazole • Gantanol		
cyclosporine	May reduce action of cyclosporine. May increase risk of nephrotoxicity.	• Monitor cyclosporine level. • Monitor renal function test results.
methotrexate	May increase bone marrow suppression.	• Monitor hematologic studies closely.
oral anticoagulants	May enhance anticoagulant effects.	• Monitor PT and INR. • Monitor patient for bleeding.
oral antidiabetics, including sulfonylureas	May enhance hypoglycemic effects.	• Monitor serum glucose level closely. • Monitor patient carefully for signs of hypoglycemia, including dizziness, headache, diaphoresis, confusion, and tachycardia. • Dosage adjustment may be needed.
PABA	May antagonize sulfonamide effects.	• Don't use together.
trimethoprim or pyrimethamine (folic acid antagonists with different mechanisms of action)	May result in synergistic antibacterial effects and delay or prevent bacterial resistance.	• This is a clinical therapeutic advantage in the treatment of malaria and toxoplasmosis.
dong quai St. John's wort	May increase risk of photosensitivity.	• Advise patient to avoid unprotected exposure to sunlight.
sun exposure	May cause photosensitivity reactions.	• Advise patient to use sunblock.
sulfasalazine • Azulfidine, Azulfidine En-tabs		
antacids	May increase systemic absorption and hazard of toxicity.	• Monitor patient for increased adverse effects, including dizziness, drowsiness, headache, altered mental status, abdominal pain, anorexia, nausea, and vomiting.

antibiotics that alter intestinal flora	May interfere with conversion of sulfasalazine to sulfapyridine and 5-aminosalicylic acid, decreasing its effectiveness.	• Monitor patient for clinical effects.
digoxin folic acid	Sulfasalazine may reduce GI absorption of these drugs.	• Monitor serum digoxin level. • Monitor patient for clinical effects.
methotrexate	May increase bone marrow suppression.	• Monitor hematologic studies closely.
oral anticoagulants	May enhance anticoagulant effects.	• Monitor PT and INR. • Monitor patient for bleeding.
oral antidiabetics, including sulfonylureas	May enhance hypoglycemic effects.	• Monitor serum glucose level closely. • Monitor patient carefully for signs of hypoglycemia, including dizziness, headache, diaphoresis, confusion, and tachycardia. • Dosage adjustment may be needed.
urine acidifying agents (such as ammonium chloride and ascorbic acid)	May increase risk of crystalluria.	• Monitor patient closely for adverse effects. • Less soluble sulfonamides such as sulfadiazine or sulfapyridine may be substituted.
dong quai feverfew garlic ginger horse chestnut red clover	May increase risk of bleeding.	• Discourage use together.
sun exposure	Photosensitivity may occur.	• Advise patient to use sunblock.

INTERACTING AGENTS	POSSIBLE EFFECTS	NURSING CONSIDERATIONS
sulindac • Clinoril		
antacids	May delay and decrease the absorption of sulindac.	• Give drugs at separate times.
anticoagulants thrombolytics	May be potentiated by the platelet-inhibiting effect of sulindac.	• Monitor PT and INR closely.
aspirin diflunisal	May decrease plasma levels of the active sulfide metabolite.	• Don't use together, if possible. • Monitor patient for reduced clinical effects of sulindac.
dimethyl sulfoxide	May decrease plasma levels of the active sulfide metabolite. Peripheral neuropathies have also been reported.	• Don't use together.
GI-irritating drugs (including antibiotics, NSAIDs, steroids)	May potentiate the adverse GI effects of sulindac.	• Monitor patient for increased GI complaints, abdominal pain, nausea, and melena.
highly protein-bound drugs (such as phenytoin, sulfonylureas, warfarin)	May cause displacement of either drug and adverse effects.	• Monitor patient for expected clinical effects and signs of toxicity for both drugs.
lithium methotrexate	May increase serum lithium level and decrease lithium clearance. May increase serum methotrexate level.	• For lithium, monitor patient for signs of toxicity, including sedation, confusion, tremors, muscle weakness, increased deep tendon reflexes, visual changes, and nystagmus. • For methotrexate, monitor patient for myelosuppression, anemia, nausea, vomiting, diarrhea, dermatitis, alopecia, melena, and fatigue.

| probenecid | May increase serum level of sulindac. Sulindac may decrease the uricosuric effect of probenecid. | • Monitor serum levels of these drugs.
• Monitor patient for toxicity.
• Dosage adjustment may be needed. |

sumatriptan succinate • Imitrex

ergot ergot derivatives	May prolong vasospastic effects.	• These drugs shouldn't be used within 24 hr of sumatriptan therapy.
MAO inhibitors	May increase effects of sumatriptan; increases risk of cardiac toxicity.	• Don't use together or within 2 wk of discontinuing MAO inhibitor therapy. • If necessary to use selective 5-HT₁ receptor agonists together, use naratriptan, which has fewer adverse reactions with MAO inhibitors.
SSRIs (citalopram, fluoxetine, fluvoxamine, nefazodone, paroxetine, sertraline, venlafaxine) sibutramine	May increase risk of serotonin syndrome (altered mental status; increased muscle tone, weakness, twitching; hyperthermia; delirium; coma; death).	• Don't use together. • If unavoidable, initial dosages may be lower, and patient must be closely monitored.
horehound	May enhance serotonergic effects.	• Advise patient not to use together. • Advise patient to consult health care provider before taking herbal preparations.

tacrolimus (FK506) • Prograf

| bromocriptine
cimetidine
clarithromycin
clotrimazole
cyclosporine
danazol
diltiazem
erythromycin | These drugs may inhibit the CYP3A enzyme system, decreasing the metabolism of tacrolimus and increasing its serum level. | • Monitor serum tacrolimus level.
• Monitor patient for increased adverse effects, including headache, paresthesia, hypertension, edema, abdominal pain, nausea, vomiting, diarrhea, hematologic and renal toxicity, electrolyte disturbances, dyspnea, and rash.
• Drug shouldn't be taken with grapefruit juice. |

(continued)

Interacting agents in **bold type** indicate severe, well-documented interactions.   †Canadian

INTERACTING AGENTS	POSSIBLE EFFECTS	NURSING CONSIDERATIONS
tacrolimus (FK506) *(continued)*		
fluconazole grapefruit juice itraconazole ketoconazole methylprednisolone metoclopramide nicardipine verapamil		
carbamazepine phenobarbital phenytoin rifabutin rifampin	These drugs may induce the CYP3A enzyme system, increasing the metabolism of tacrolimus with a resulting decrease in serum level.	• Monitor tacrolimus level. • Monitor effectiveness of tacrolimus.
cyclosporine	May increase risk of excess nephrotoxicity.	• Don't give together. • When changing therapy, give tacrolimus at least 24 hr after last cyclosporine dose.
immunosuppressants (except adrenal corticosteroids)	May oversuppress immune system.	• Monitor patient closely, especially during times of stress.
live-virus vaccines	May interfere with immune response to live-virus vaccines.	• Avoid giving routine immunizations.
nephrotoxic drugs (such as aminoglycosides, amphotericin B, cisplatin, cyclosporine)	May cause additive or synergistic effects.	• Avoid use together, if possible. • If used together, monitor renal function test results and serum drug levels. • Don't give with cyclosporine.
food	May inhibit drug absorption.	• Give drug on empty stomach.

tamoxifen citrate • Nolvadex, Nolvadex-D†, Tamofen†

antacids	May affect absorption of enteric-coated tablet.	• Give drugs 2 hr apart.
bromocriptine	May increase tamoxifen level.	• Monitor patient for increased adverse effects. • Dosage adjustment may be needed.
coumadin	May cause significant increase in anticoagulation effect.	• Monitor PT and INR. • Dose adjustment may be needed.
cytotoxic drugs	May increase thromboembolic events.	• Assess patient for thrombembolic risk factors. Monitor patient for leg pain, redness, swelling, chest pain, and shortness of breath.
estrogens	May decrease therapeutic effect of drug.	• Monitor patient for clinical effects. • Dose adjustment may be needed.

tamsulosin hydrochloride • Flomax

alpha blockers	May interact with tamsulosin.	• Don't use together.
cimetidine	May decrease clearance of tamsulosin.	• Monitor patient for increased adverse effects, including dizziness, headache, hypotension, and increased risk of infection.

telmisartan • Micardis

digoxin	May increase serum digoxin level.	• Monitor digoxin level. • Monitor patient for signs of digoxin toxicity, including fatigue, asthenia, dizziness, arrhythmias, visual disturbances, nausea, vomiting, and diarrhea.
warfarin	May slightly decrease plasma warfarin level.	• Monitor PT and INR.
potassium-containing salt substitutes	May increase risk of hyperkalemia.	• Advise patient to avoid using together.

Interacting agents in **bold type** indicate severe, well-documented interactions.   †Canadian   **267**

INTERACTING AGENTS	POSSIBLE EFFECTS	NURSING CONSIDERATIONS

temazepam • Restoril

alcohol calendula CNS depressants hops kava lemon balm passionflower skullcap valerian	May increase CNS depression.	• Use together cautiously. • Monitor patient for increased sedation, headache, dizziness, agitation, asthenia, and respiratory depression. • Advise patient to avoid alcohol. • Advise patient against concomitant herbal use. • Advise patient to contact health care professional before using any herbal preparations.

tetracycline hydrochloride • Achromycin, Ala-Tet, Novotetra†, Robitet, Sumycin, Teline, Tetralan†, Topicycline

antacids containing aluminum, calcium, magnesium magnesium-containing laxatives **oral iron** sodium bicarbonate dairy products milk food	May decrease absorption of tetracycline.	• Separate administration times by 3 to 4 hr. • May give enteric-coated or sustained-release iron preparations with tetracycline. • Should give antibiotic 1 hr before or 2 hr after food and dairy products.
anticoagulants	May enhance anticoagulation effects.	• Monitor PT and INR. • Dosage adjustment may be needed.
cimetidine	May decrease GI absorption of tetracycline.	• Monitor patient's clinical response. • Dosage adjustment of tetracycline may be needed.
digoxin	May increase digoxin level.	• Monitor digoxin level. • Signs of digoxin toxicity include fatigue, asthenia, dizziness, arrhythmias, visual

	disturbances, nausea, vomiting, and diarrhea.
	• Dosage adjustment may be needed.

methoxyflurane	May increase risk of nephrotoxicity.	• Don't use together.
oral contraceptives	May decrease contraceptive effect.	• Advise patient to use another contraceptive method.
penicillin	May inhibit cell growth from bacteriostatic action.	• Avoid giving these drugs together. • If unavoidable, give penicillin 2 to 3 hr before tetracycline. • Monitor patient for expected clinical effects.
sun exposure	May enhance photosensitivity reactions.	• Advise patient to use sunblock.

thalidomide • Thalomid

alcohol barbiturates chlorpromazine reserpine	May enhance sedative activity.	• Monitor patient for increased drowsiness and somnolence. • Advise patient to avoid alcohol.
drugs linked to peripheral neuropathy	May increase risk of peripheral neuropathy.	• Monitor patient for increased pain, numbness, and tingling in the extremities.
drugs that may reduce efficacy of hormonal contraception (carbamazepine, griseofulvin, HIV-protease inhibitors, phenytoin, rifabutin, rifampin)	May increase potential for thalidomide-induced teratogenicity if pregnancy occurs.	• Patient must be advised to use 2 other highly effective methods of barrier contraception.
food	May decrease absorption of drug.	• Give drug 1 hr after meals.

Interacting agents in **bold type** indicate severe, well documented interactions.   †Canadian

INTERACTING AGENTS	POSSIBLE EFFECTS	NURSING CONSIDERATIONS
theophylline • Accurbron†, Aerolate, Aquaphyllin, Asmalix†, Bronkodyl†, Elixomin†, Elixophyllin†, Lanophyllin†, Slo-Phyllin, Theoclear-80, Theolair Liquid, Theostat 80† (immediate-release liquids); Bronkodyl, Elixophyllin, Quibron-T Dividose, Slo-Phyllin (immediate-release tablets and capsules); Quibron-T/SR, Respbid, Sustaire, Theochron, Theo-Dur, Theolair-SR, Theo-Sav, Theo-Time, T-Phyl, Uni-Dur, Uniphyl; Aerolate, Elixophyllin, Slo-bid Gyrocaps, Slo-Phyllin, Theobid Duracaps, Theochron, Theoclear L.A., Theo-Dur Sprinkle, Theospan-SR, Theo-24, Theovent Long-Acting (timed-release capsules)		
adenosine	May decrease antiarrhythmic effectiveness.	• Monitor ECG for clinical effect. • Higher doses of adenosine may be needed.
allopurinol cacao tree caffeine calcium channel blockers **cimetidine** disulfiram influenza virus vaccine interferon **macrolide antibiotics (such as erythromycin)** methotrexate oral contraceptives quinolone antibiotics (such as ciprofloxacin) thiabendazole ticlodipine zileuton	May decrease hepatic clearance of theophylline; may elevate theophylline level.	• Monitor serum theophylline level closely; dosage adjustment may be needed, to avoid toxicity. Signs of toxicity include tachycardia, nausea, vomiting, diarrhea, restlessness, headaches, agitation, palpitations, and arrhythmias. • Advise patient against concomitant herbal use. • Advise patient to contact health care professional before using any herbal preparations. • Advise patient to avoid or limit caffeine use.
barbiturates **nicotine** phenytoin rifampin St. John's wort	May enhance metabolism and decrease theophylline serum level.	• Monitor patient for decreased effect. • Dosage adjustments may be needed. • Advise patient against concomitant herbal or nicotine use. • Advise patient to contact health care professional before using any herbal preparations.

beta blockers (especially nadolol and propranolol)	May cause antagonism. May cause bronchospasm in sensitive patients.	• Monitor patient for worsened clinical status. • Alternatively, beta-selective drugs may be used.
carbamazepine isoniazid loop diuretics	May increase or decrease theophylline level.	• Monitor serum theophylline level. • Monitor patient for loss of clinical effects or increased adverse effects and toxicity.
charcoal	May reduce absorption and removal of drug from systemic circulation.	• Don't use charcoal as an antidiarrheal in patients taking theophylline.
ephedrine sympathomimetics	May exhibit synergistic toxicity with these drugs, predisposing patient to arrhythmias.	• Limit concomitant use. • Monitor serum theophylline and potassium levels. • Monitor vital signs and ECG.
halothane	May increase risk of arrhythmias.	• Don't use together.
thioamines thyroid hormones	Theophylline clearance may increase in hyperthyroid state and decrease in hypothyroid state.	• Monitor thyroid studies and theophylline level. • Monitor patient for euthyroid state.
lithium	May increase lithium excretion.	• Monitor serum lithium level. • Monitor patient for clinical effect.
cayenne ipriflavone	May increase risk of theophylline toxicity.	• Advise patient against concomitant use. • Advise patient to contact health care professional before using any herbs. • Monitor serum theophylline level.
guarana	May cause additive CNS and CV effects.	• Advise patient against concomitant use. • Advise patient to contact health care professional before using any herbal preparations.

(continued)

Interacting agents in **bold type** indicate severe, well documented interactions.   †Canadian

INTERACTING AGENTS	POSSIBLE EFFECTS	NURSING CONSIDERATIONS
theophylline (continued)		
food	May accelerate release of theophylline from extended-release products.	• Tell patient to take Theo-24 on an empty stomach.
smoking	May increase elimination of theophylline, increasing dosage requirements.	• Discourage smoking. • Monitor theophylline response and serum level. • If patient is a smoker and has a stable theophylline level, then quits smoking, he should notify his prescriber to have his theophylline level assessed and possibly his dosage reduced.
thiabendazole • Mintezol		
theophylline	May increase risk of theophylline toxicity.	• Monitor serum theophylline level closely; dosage adjustment may be needed, to avoid toxicity. Signs of toxicity include tachycardia, nausea, vomiting, diarrhea, restlessness, headaches, agitation, palpitations, and arrhythmias.
tiagabine hydrochloride • Gabitril		
carbamazepine phenobarbital phenytoin	May increase tiagabine clearance.	• Monitor serum tiagabine level. • Monitor patient for adequately controlled seizures.
alcohol CNS depressants	May enhance CNS effects.	• Monitor patient for increased sedation, dizziness, headache, agitation, asthenia, and respiratory depression. • Advise patient to avoid alcohol.

ticarcillin disodium • Ticar

lithium	May alter renal elimination of lithium.	• Monitor serum lithium level closely.
methotrexate	Large doses of ticarcillin may interfere with renal tubular secretion of methotrexate, delaying elimination and prolonging elevated serum level of methotrexate.	• Monitor patient for methotrexate toxicity; monitor serum level. • An alternative antibiotic may be needed.
oral contraceptives	May decrease efficacy of oral contraceptives.	• Advise patient to use barrier contraception during penicillin therapy.
probenecid	May increase serum level of ticarcillin and other penicillins.	• Probenecid may be used for this purpose.
tetracyclines	May reduce ticarcillin effectiveness.	• Avoid using together.

ticlopidine hydrochloride • Ticlid

antacids	May decrease serum level of ticlopidine.	• Separate administration times by at least 2 hr.
aspirin	May potentiate effects of aspirin on platelets.	• Concomitant use is not recommended.
cimetidine	May decrease clearance of ticlopidine; may increase toxicity risk.	• Don't use together.
digoxin	May cause slightly decreased serum digoxin level.	• Monitor serum digoxin level.
hydantoins	May inhibit hepatic metabolism of hydantoins.	• Monitor serum hydantoin level. • Monitor patient for signs of toxicity, including drowsiness, confusion or decreased level of consciousness, nausea, vomiting, nystagmus, ataxia, dysarthia,

(continued)

Interacting agents in **bold type** indicate severe, well documented interactions.   †Canadian

INTERACTING AGENTS	POSSIBLE EFFECTS	NURSING CONSIDERATIONS
ticlopidine hydrochloride *(continued)*		
hydantoins *(continued)*		tremor, slurred speech, hypotension, arrhythmias, and respiratory depression.
theophylline	May increase risk of theophylline toxicity.	• Monitor serum theophylline level. • Monitor patient for signs of toxicity, including nausea, vomiting, insomnia, irritability, tachycardia, arrhythmias, tachypnea, and seizures. • Dosage adjustment may be needed.
red clover	May increase risk of bleeding.	• Advise patient not to use together. • Advise patient to consult health care provider before taking any herbal preparations.
timolol maleate • Apo-Timol†, Blocadren		
cardiac glycosides diltiazem **verapamil**	May cause excessive bradycardia and increase depressant effect on myocardium.	• Monitor cardiac function. • Dosage adjustment may be needed.
catecholamine-depleting drugs (such as reserpine)	May have additive effect when given with beta blockers.	• Monitor patient for hypotension and bradycardia.
clonidine	May cause life-threatening hypertension.	• Monitor patient's BP closely when these drugs are used together and after one is stopped.
epinephrine	May increase potential for hypertensive episode followed by bradycardia.	• The beta blocker should be stopped 3 days before anticipated epinephrine use. • Don't use together. • Monitor BP.

ergot alkaloids	May increase potential for peripheral ischemia or gangrene.	• Monitor patient for peripheral ischemia (cold extremities). • Dosages may need adjustment or drugs may need to be stopped.
indomethacin	May decrease antihypertensive effect.	• Monitor BP. • Dosage adjustment may be needed.
insulin oral antidiabetics	May alter requirements for these drugs in previously stabilized diabetic patients.	• Monitor serum glucose level closely. Monitor patient carefully for signs of hypoglycemia, including dizziness, headache, diaphoresis, confusion, and tachycardia. • Dosage adjustment may be needed.
quinidine	May increase beta blocker effect.	• Monitor BP and HR. • Dosage adjustment may be needed.
theophylline	May increase serum theophylline level. May reduce effects of both drugs.	• Monitor serum theophylline level closely. • Dosage adjustment may be needed. • Signs of toxicity include tachycardia, nausea, vomiting, diarrhea, restlessness, headaches, agitation, palpitations, and arrhythmias. • Monitor patient for clinical effects of both drugs.

tolazamide • Tolinase

beta blockers (including ophthalmics)	May increase risk of hypoglycemia, mask its symptoms (increasing pulse rate and BP), and prolong it by blocking gluconeogenesis.	• Monitor serum glucose level closely. • Monitor patient carefully for signs of hypoglycemia, including dizziness, headache, diaphoresis, confusion, and tachycardia. • Dosage adjustment may be needed.

(continued)

INTERACTING AGENTS	POSSIBLE EFFECTS	NURSING CONSIDERATIONS
tolazamide (continued)		
calcium channel blockers corticosteroids estrogens isoniazid phenothiazines sympathomimetics oral contraceptives phenytoin thiazide diuretics triamterene thyroid hormones	May decrease hypoglycemic effect	• Monitor serum glucose level. • Monitor patient for signs of hyper-glycemia (fatigue, polyuria, polydipsia, dehydration, electrolyte disturbances, weight loss, abdominal pain, altered mental status, tachycardia, hypotension, glucosuria, ketonuria). • Dosage adjustment may be needed.
NSAIDs chloramphenicol insulin MAO inhibitors probenecid salicylates sulfonamides	May enhance hypoglycemic effect.	• Monitor serum glucose level closely. • Monitor patient carefully for signs of hypoglycemia, including dizziness, headache, diaphoresis, confusion, and tachycardia. • Dosage adjustment may be needed.
oral anticoagulants	May increase hypoglycemic activity or enhance anticoagulant effect.	• Monitor serum glucose level and PT and INR.
alcohol	May cause disulfiram-like reaction (nausea, vomiting, abdominal cramps, headaches).	• Advise patient to avoid alcohol.
tolbutamide • Orinase		
anticoagulants	May increase hypoglycemic activity and enhance anticoagulant effect.	• Monitor blood glucose levels, PT, and INR. • Dosage adjustment may be needed.

beta blockers (including ophthalmics)	May mask symptoms of hypoglycemia and prolong hypoglycemia.	• Monitor serum glucose closely. Monitor patient carefully for signs of hypoglycemia, including dizziness, headache, diaphoresis, confusion, and tachycardia. • Dosage adjustment may be needed.
calcium channel blockers corticosteroids estrogens isoniazid oral contraceptives phenothiazines phenytoin sympathomimetics thiazide diuretics thyroid hormones triamterene	May decrease hypoglycemic effect.	• Monitor serum glucose level. • Monitor patient for signs of hyperglycemia (fatigue, polyuria, polydipsia, dehydration, electrolyte disturbances, weight loss, abdominal pain, altered mental status, tachycardia, hypotension, glucosuria, ketonuria). • Dosage adjustment may be needed.
chloramphenicol insulin MAO inhibitors NSAIDs **phenylbutazones** probenecid salicylates sulfonamides	May enhance hypoglycemic effect.	• Monitor serum glucose level closely. • Monitor patient carefully for signs of hypoglycemia, including dizziness, headache, diaphoresis, confusion, and tachycardia. • Dosage adjustment may be needed.
aloe bilberry leaf bitter melon burdock dandelion fenugreek garlic ginseng	May improve serum glucose control, requiring a reduction of antidiabetics.	• Advise patient to discuss the use of herbal medicines with prescriber before use.

Interacting agents in **bold type** indicate severe, well documented interactions.   †Canadian

INTERACTING AGENTS	POSSIBLE EFFECTS	NURSING CONSIDERATIONS
tolbutamide (continued)		
alcohol	May produce a disulfiram-like reaction with nausea, vomiting, abdominal cramps, and headaches.	• Advise patient to avoid alcohol.
tolcapone • Tasmar		
desipramine	May increase risk of adverse effects.	• Monitor patient closely for increased adverse effects.
MAO inhibitors	Hypertensive crisis may occur.	• Avoid use together.
tolterodine tartrate • Detrol		
azole antifungals cytochrome P450 3A4 inhibitors	May elevate tolterodine plasma level, increasing adverse effects.	• Don't give tolterodine doses above 1 mg b.i.d. with these drugs.
fluoxetine	May increase tolterodine level.	• Monitor patient for increased adverse effects. • Dosage adjustments are not usually needed.
tramadol hydrochloride • Ultram		
carbamazepine	May increase tramadol metabolism.	• Monitor patient closely for clinical effect. • Dose adjustment may be needed.
alcohol CNS depressants	May cause additive effects.	• Monitor patient closely for increased sedation, dizziness, ataxia, tremor, agitation, and respiratory depression. • Tramadol dose may need to be reduced. • Advise patient to avoid alcohol.
MAO inhibitors	May increase risk of seizures.	• Monitor patient closely for adverse effects.

neuroleptics

- Avoid giving this combination in patients at risk for seizures.

trastuzumab • Herceptin

anthracyclines	May increase risk of cardiotoxicity.	• Monitor patient for signs of cardiotoxicity, including dyspnea, increased cough, paroxysmal nocturnal dyspnea, peripheral edema, murmurs (S_3 gallop), cardiomyopathy, congestive heart failure, and reduced ejection fraction.
paclitaxel	May increase trastuzumab serum level.	• Monitor patient for increased adverse effects, including nausea, vomiting, diarrhea, cardiotoxicity, anemia, leukopenia, pancytopenia, pain, rash, increased risk of infection, and increased risk of infusion reaction.

tretinoin (topical) • Renova, Retin-A, Retin-A Micro

skin preparations containing alcohol abrasive cleaners medicated cosmetics topical agents	May increase risk of skin irritation.	• Advise patient to use these agents with caution. • Monitor patient's skin integrity; observe skin for redness, excessive drying, and chafing.
sun exposure	May cause photosensitivity reactions.	• Advise patient to avoid prolonged or unprotected exposure to the sun.

triamterene • Dyrenium

antihypertensives	May enhance hypotension.	• Monitor BP. • May be used for a therapeutic advantage.
cimetidine	May increase bioavailability of triamterene.	• Monitor patient for increased adverse effects.

(continued)

INTERACTING AGENTS	POSSIBLE EFFECTS	NURSING CONSIDERATIONS
triamterene *(continued)*		
cimetidine *(continued)*		• Triamterene dose may need to be reduced or cimetidine stopped.
lithium	May decrease lithium clearance.	• Avoid use together.
ACE inhibitors (such as captopril and enalapril) potassium-sparing diuretics **potassium supplements** potassium-containing drugs (such as parenteral penicillin G) potassium-containing salt substitutes potassium-rich foods	May increase risk of hyperkalemia.	• Monitor renal function and serum potassium level. Monitor patient for signs of hyperkalemia, including mental confusion, neuromuscular excitability, weakness, paresthesia, ascending flaccid paralysis, and cardiac abnormalities (peaked T waves, depressed ST segment, absence of P wave, prolonged QT interval, and widened QRS complex). • Advise patient to avoid salt substitutes containing potassium.
NSAIDs	May alter potassium excretion.	• Monitor renal function test results and serum potassium level.
sun exposure	May cause photosensitivity reactions.	• Advise patient to avoid excessive sun exposure.
triazolam • Halcion		
antidepressants antihistamines barbiturates general anesthetics MAO inhibitors narcotics phenothiazines	May enhance CNS-depressant effects.	• Monitor patient closely for signs of increased CNS depression, including increased sedation, headache, dizziness, ataxia, confusion, agitation, and respiratory depression. • Dose reduction of triazolam or extended dosing interval may be needed.

azole antifungal drugs (such as fluconazole, itraconazole, **ketoconazole**, miconazole)	May increase serum levels. May prolong CNS effects and psychomotor impairment.	• Don't use triazolam with ketoconazole or itraconazole. • If triazolam is used with other drugs, the triazolam dose may need to be reduced.
cimetidine disulfiram grapefruit juice isoniazid oral contraceptives	May increase plasma triazolam level.	• Monitor patient for increased sedation. • Dose reduction of triazolam or extended dosing interval may be needed. • Don't give drug with grapefruit juice.
erythromycin	May decrease triazolam clearance.	• Monitor patient for increased sedation. • Dose reduction of triazolam or extended dosing interval may be needed.
haloperidol	May decrease serum level of haloperidol.	• Monitor patient closely for clinical effect.
levodopa	May decrease therapeutic effects of levodopa.	• Monitor patient for clinical effects. • Triazolam may need to be stopped.
indinavir non-nucleoside reverse transcriptase inhibitors (such as delavirdine and efavirenz) ritonavir	May increase sedation and respiratory depression.	• Don't use together.
catnip kava lady's slipper lemon balm passionflower sassafras skullcap valerian	Sedative effects may be enhanced.	• Discourage using together. • Advise patient to consult health care provider before using any herbal preparations.

(continued)

INTERACTING AGENTS	POSSIBLE EFFECTS	NURSING CONSIDERATIONS
triazolam *(continued)*		
alcohol	May enhance amnesia and cause excessive CNS depression.	• Advise patient to avoid alcohol.
smoking (heavy)	May lower triazolam effectiveness.	• Discourage smoking.
trimethoprim • Proloprim, Trimpex		
dapsone	May increase serum levels of both drugs.	• Monitor patient for toxicity.
phenytoin	May increase serum phenytoin level.	• Monitor phenytoin level. Monitor patient for signs of phenytoin toxicity, including drowsiness, confusion, or decreased level of consciousness, nausea, vomiting, nystagmus, ataxia, dysarthria, tremor, slurred speech, hypotension, arrhythmias, and respiratory depression.
dong quai St. John's wort	May increase risk of photosensitivity.	• Advise patient to use sunblock.
methotrexate	May increase risk of bone marrow suppression and megaloblastic anemia.	• Avoid use together, if possible. • If used together, monitor patient for hematologic toxicity.
trovafloxacin mesylate • Trovan Tablets **alatrofloxacin mesylate** • Trovan I.V.		
aluminum-, magnesium-, and iron-containing preparations (such as antacids and vitamin-minerals; and divalent and trivalent cations, such as didanosine) sucralfate	May reduce oral bioavailability of drug.	• Separate administration times of oral trovafloxacin and any of these drugs by at least 2 hr.

morphine (I.V.)	May reduce trovafloxacin plasma level.	• Give I.V. morphine at least 2 hr after oral trovafloxacin in fasting state and at least 4 hr after oral trovafloxacin is taken with food.
warfarin	May enhance anticoagulation effect.	• Monitor PT and INR.
sun exposure	May increase photosensitivity reaction.	• Advise patient to use sunblock.

urokinase • Abbokinase, Abbokinase Open-Cath

aminocaproic acid	May inhibit urokinase-induced activation of plasminogen.	• Avoid use together.
anticoagulants (including heparin and oral anticoagulants)	May increase risk of hemorrhage.	• Heparin must be stopped and its effects allowed to diminish. • It may also be necessary to reverse effects of oral anticoagulants before beginning therapy. • If heparin is used during intracoronary urokinase administration, monitor patient closely for increased bleeding and monitor PTT.
dong quai feverfew garlic ginger horse chestnut red clover	May increase risk of bleeding.	• Discourage use together.
aspirin drugs affecting platelet activity indomethacin phenylbutazone	May increase risk of bleeding.	• Avoid use together.

INTERACTING AGENTS	POSSIBLE EFFECTS	NURSING CONSIDERATIONS
valacyclovir hydrochloride • Valtrex		
cimetidine probenecid	May reduce rate, but not extent, of conversion of valacyclovir to acyclovir. May reduce renal clearance of acyclovir, increasing acyclovir blood level.	• Monitor patient for potential increased adverse effects. • Dosage adjustment may be needed; no dosage adjustment is usually needed in patients with normal renal function.
valproic acid • Depakene, Epival† **divalproex sodium** • Depakote, Depakote ER, Depakote Sprinkle **valproate sodium** • Depacon		
carbamazepine	May decrease valproic acid level. May alter carbamazepine level.	• Monitor serum drug level. • Monitor patient for signs of toxicity and loss of seizure control.
clonazepam	May cause absence seizures and severe drowsiness.	• Monitor patient for loss of seizure control and severe drowsiness.
felbamate salicylates	May increase valproate level.	• Monitor valproate level. • Monitor patient for signs of toxicity, including tremor, drowsiness, ataxia, nystagmus, changes in personality, and elevated liver enzymes. • Dosage adjustments may be needed.
lamotrigine	May increase lamotrigine level.	• Monitor patient for signs of toxicity, including dizziness, headache, somnolence, and decreased level of consciousness. • Dosage adjustments may be needed.
CNS antidepressants MAO inhibitors	May potentiate effects of these drugs.	• Monitor patient for increased adverse effects.

oral anticoagulants		• Monitor patient for increased sedation, headache, dizziness, agitation, asthenia, and respiratory depression. • Monitor PT and INR. • Dosage adjustments may be needed.
phenobarbital phenytoin primidone	May increase serum levels of these drugs. May cause excessive somnolence.	• Monitor serum drug levels. • Monitor patient for increased somnolence. • Dosage adjustments may be needed.
alcohol	May decrease valproic acid effectiveness. May increase CNS adverse effects.	• Discourage use together.

vancomycin hydrochloride • Vancocin, Vancoled

aminoglycosides amphotericin b capreomycin cisplatin colistin methoxyflurane polymyxin B	May increase additive effect on these drugs.	• Monitor renal function test results and serum drug levels if appropriate. • Perform a baseline hearing test and monitor periodically thereafter. • Dosage adjustments may be needed.
nondepolarizing muscle relaxants	May enhance neuromuscular blockade.	• Use together only if needed. • Monitor neuromuscular function; careful titration is needed. • Mechanical respiratory support measures should be available.

vasopressin • Pitressin Synthetic

carbamazepine chlorpropamide clofibrate	May potentiate vasopressin's antidiuretic effect.	• Monitor patient for increased clinical effects and signs of water intoxication, including drowsiness, listlessness,

(continued)

Interacting agents in **bold type** indicate severe, well-documented interactions.   †Canadian

INTERACTING AGENTS	POSSIBLE EFFECTS	NURSING CONSIDERATIONS
vasopressin *(continued)*		
fludrocortisone phenformin TCAs urea		headache, confusion, anuria, and weight gain.
alcohol demeclocycline epinephrine heparin lithium norepinephrine	May decrease antidiuretic effect.	• Monitor patient for expected clinical effects. • Advise patient to avoid alcohol.
venlafaxine hydrochloride • Effexor, Effexor XR		
cimetidine CNS-active drugs	May cause pronounced increase in venlafaxine level in elderly patients and in those with hepatic dysfunction or preexisting hypertension.	• Use cautiously. • Monitor patient for increased adverse effects and signs of toxicity, including somnolence, seizures, and prolongation of the QT interval.
MAO inhibitors sibutramine sumatriptan	May precipitate a syndrome similar to neuroleptic malignant syndrome.	• Don't start venlafaxine within 14 days of stopping an MAO inhibitor; don't start MAO inhibitor within 7 days of stopping venlafaxine. • Avoid using with sibutramine or sumatriptan; if unavoidable, use lower dosages initially and monitor patient closely.
yohimbé	May cause additive stimulation.	• Advise patient to use together cautiously. • Advise patient to consult health care provider before taking herbal preparations.

beta blockers	May have additive effects leading to heart failure, conduction disturbances, arrhythmias, and hypotension, especially if high beta-blocker doses are used, if drugs are given I.V., or if patient has moderately severe to severe heart failure, severe cardiomyopathy, or recent MI.	• Monitor cardiac status (vital signs, ECG) closely. • Decreased dosages may be needed.
carbamazepine	May increase serum carbamazepine level and subsequent toxicity.	• Use together cautiously. • Monitor for signs of toxicity, including dizziness, ataxia, respiratory depression, arrhythmias, BP changes, impaired consciousness, restlessness, abnormal reflexes, seizures, nausea, vomiting, and urinary retention.
cyclosporine	May increase serum level of cyclosporine.	• Monitor therapeutic effect. • Dosage adjustment of cyclosporine may be needed.
digoxin	May increase serum digoxin level by 50% to 75% during first week of therapy.	• Monitor serum digoxin level. • Monitor patient for signs of digoxin toxicity, including fatigue, asthenia, dizziness, arrhythmias, visual disturbances, nausea, vomiting, and diarrhea. • Dosage adjustments may be needed.
disopyramide	May combine negative inotropic effects.	• Don't give disopyramide less than 48 hr before and less than 24 hr after verapamil.
flecainide	May add to negative inotropic effect and prolong AV conduction.	• Use together cautiously. • Monitor cardiac status.

(continued)

Interacting agents in **bold type** indicate severe, well-documented interactions.   †Canadian

INTERACTING AGENTS	POSSIBLE EFFECTS	NURSING CONSIDERATIONS
verapamil hydrochloride *(continued)*		
inhalation anesthetics	May cause excessive CV depression.	• Monitor patient's vital signs and respiratory status closely; titrate drugs carefully to avoid CV compromise.
lithium	May increase sensitivity of lithium effects.	• Monitor patient for increased adverse effects. • Lithium dosage adjustments may be needed.
neuromuscular blockers	Verapamil may potentiate the action of these drugs.	• Monitor vital signs and respiratory status closely. • Dosage of one or both drugs may need to be reduced.
antihypertensives drugs that attenuate alpha-adrenergic response (such as methyldopa, prazosin) quinidine (to treat hypertrophic cardiomyopathy)	May cause hypotension. Use of verapamil with quinidine may produce bradycardia, ventricular tachycardia, or AV block.	• Monitor BP closely. • Dosage adjustment may be needed. • Don't use quinidine and verapamil together.
phenobarbital	May increase verapamil clearance.	• Monitor patient for clinical response.
rifampin	May substantially reduce verapamil's oral bioavailability.	• Monitor patient for therapeutic effects. • Dosage adjustments may be needed. • I.V. verapamil may be used instead of the oral form. • Verapamil dose may need to be adjusted after rifampin is stopped.
theophylline	May increase serum theophylline level.	• Monitor serum theophylline level. Monitor patient for signs of toxicity, including

		nausea, vomiting, insomnia, irritability, tachycardia, arrhythmias, tachypnea, and seizures. • Dosage adjustment may be needed.
yerba maté	May decrease clearance of yerba maté methylxanthines and cause toxicity.	• Advise patient to avoid using together. • Advise patient to consult health care provider before taking herbal preparations.
food	May increase absorption.	• Advise patient to take drug with food.
alcohol	May prolong intoxication effect.	• Advise patient to avoid alcohol.

vinblastine sulfate (VLB) • Velban, Velbet†

azole antifungal drugs erythromycin	May cause toxicity of vinblastine.	• Don't use together. • If used together, monitor patient for signs of toxicity, including stomatitis, ileus, constipation, mental depression, paresthesia, myalgia, loss of deep reflexes, and myelosuppression. • Vinblastine dose may need to be reduced or anti-infective drug stopped.
mitomycin	May cause acute shortness of breath and severe bronchospasm.	• If used together, monitor patient's respiratory status closely.
phenytoin	May result in a lower serum phenytoin level.	• Monitor phenytoin level. • Monitor patient for loss of seizure control. • Phenytoin dosage adjustment may be needed.

INTERACTING AGENTS	POSSIBLE EFFECTS	NURSING CONSIDERATIONS
vincristine sulfate • Oncovin, Vincasar PFS		
asparaginase azole antifungal drugs	May decrease hepatic clearance of vincristine.	• Don't use with azole antifungal drugs, if possible. • If used together, monitor patient for signs of increased toxicity, including alopecia, myelosuppression, paresthesias, neuritic pain, motor difficulties, loss of deep tendon reflexes, nausea, vomiting, ileus, and constipation.
calcium channel blockers	May enhance vincristine accumulation in cells.	• Monitor patient closely for increased adverse effects. • Dosage adjustment may be needed.
digoxin	May decrease digoxin level.	• Monitor serum digoxin level.
methotrexate	May increase therapeutic effect of methotrexate.	• Monitor patient for toxicity. • A lower dosage of methotrexate may be needed.
mitomycin	May increase frequency of bronchospasm and acute pulmonary reactions.	• Monitor patient's respiratory status closely.
neurotoxic drugs	May increase neurotoxicity and additive effect.	• Monitor patient for signs of additive neurotoxicity, including muscle weakness and cramps, peripheral neuropathy, sensory loss, loss of deep tendon reflexes, paresthesia, and wristdrop and footdrop. • Dosage adjustments may be needed.
phenytoin	May decrease plasma phenytoin level.	• Monitor phenytoin level. • Monitor patient for loss of seizure control. • Phenytoin dosage adjustment may be needed.

acetaminophen	May increase bleeding with use of acetaminophen longer than 2 wk and doses > 2 g/day.	• Monitor PT and INR more frequently; limit acetaminophen use. • Warfarin dose may need to be adjusted.
alcohol allopurinol **amiodarone** **anabolic steroids** cephalosporins chloramphenicol **cimetidine** ciprofloxacin **clofibrate** **danazol** **dextrothyroxine** diazoxide diflunisal **disulfiram** **erythromycin** **glucagons** heparin ibuprofen influenza virus vaccine isoniazid **itraconazole** ketoprofen lovastatin methimazole **metronidazole** **miconazole** **nalidixic acid**	May increase hypoprothrombinemic effects via inhibition of warfarin metabolism or displacement of warfarin from plasma protein binding sites; this results in elevated PT and INR. Patient may be at risk for increased bleeding tendencies or hemorrhage.	• Don't use anabolic or androgenic steroids, cimetidine, fibric acids (clofibrate), and phenylbutazones together. • Using drugs together that increase anticoagulant effects should be done carefully with close monitoring of PT and INR during initial 1 to 2 wk of therapy and when drug is stopped. • Dosage adjustments may be needed. For example, warfarin dose may be reduced by 50% when used with amiodarone. • Monitor patient for increased bleeding tendencies (bruising, petechiae, bleeding gums, epistaxis, prolonged bleeding after injury, melena, GI bleeding, hematuria, and hematemesis). • Advise patient to avoid alcohol.

(continued)

Interacting agents in **bold type** indicate severe, well-documented interactions.   †Canadian

INTERACTING AGENTS	POSSIBLE EFFECTS	NURSING CONSIDERATIONS
warfarin sodium (continued)		
neomycin (oral) norfloxacin ofloxacin omeprazole penicillins pentoxifylline **phenylbutazones** propafenone propoxyphene propylthiouracil quinidine **salicylates** simvastatin streptokinase sulfinpyrazone **sulfonamides** sulindac tamoxifen tetracyclines thiazides **thyroid hormones** TCAs urokinase vitamin E		
anticonvulsants	May increase serum levels of phenytoin and phenobarbital.	▪ Monitor serum levels of these drugs. ▪ Monitor patient for increased adverse effects.
barbiturates	May inhibit anticoagulant effect for several wk after barbiturate withdrawal, and fa-	▪ Monitor patient closely; monitor PT and INR.

	tal hemorrhage can occur after cessation of barbiturate effect.	• If barbiturates are withdrawn, anticoagulant dose should be reduced.
carbamazepine corticosteroids ethchlorvynol **glutethimide** griseofulvin oral contraceptives **rifampin** **vitamin K**	May decrease anticoagulant effect.	• Monitor PT and INR. • Dosage adjustments may be needed when therapy starts and stops. • Assess patient's consumption of food or nutritional supplements containing vitamin K.
chloral hydrate	May increase or decrease anticoagulant effect of warfarin.	• Monitor PT and INR. • Benzodiazepines may be considered as an alternative.
ethacrynic acid indomethacin mefenamic acid **phenylbutazone** sulfinpyrazone	May increase anticoagulant effect of warfarin and cause severe GI irritation (may be ulcerogenic).	• Monitor PT and INR. • Using with phenylbutazone is not recommended. • Monitor patient for increased GI complaints, abdominal pain, melena, and increased bleeding or bruising tendencies.
cholestyramine	May decrease anticoagulant effect of warfarin.	• Give 6 hr after warfarin.
ginseng green tea St. John's wort	May decrease anticoagulant effects.	• Advise patient to avoid using together. • Advise patient to consult health care provider before taking herbal preparations.
angelica devil's claw garlic ginkgo	May increase the risk for bleeding.	• Advise patient to avoid using together. • Advise patient to consult health care provider before taking herbal preparations.
foods or enteral products containing vitamin K	May impair anticoagulation.	• Advise patient to maintain a consistent daily intake of leafy green vegetables.

Interacting agents in **bold type** indicate severe, well-documented interactions.   †Canadian

INTERACTING AGENTS	POSSIBLE EFFECTS	NURSING CONSIDERATIONS
zalcitabine (dideoxycytidine, ddC) • Hivid		
antacids containing aluminum or magnesium	May decrease absorption of zalcitabine.	• Separate administration times.
cimetidine probenecid	May decrease elimination of zalcitabine.	• Monitor patient for toxicity. • Dosage adjustments may be needed.
drugs that cause peripheral neuropathy (such as chloramphenicol, cisplatin, dapsone, didanosine, disulfiram, ethionamide, glutethimide, gold salts, hydralazine, iodoquinol, isoniazid, metronidazole, nitrofurantoin, phenytoin, ribavirin, stavudine, vincristine)	May increase risk of peripheral neuropathy.	• Don't use with didanosine and stavudine. • Monitor patient for signs of peripheral neuropathy, including loss of sensation, muscle atrophy, weakness, diminished reflexes, pain, and paresthesia. • If patient has history of peripheral neuropathy, alternative drug therapy may be considered.
drugs that may impair renal function (aminoglycosides, amphotericin, foscarnet)	May increase risk of zalcitabine-induced adverse effects.	• Limit concomitant use. • Monitor patient for increased adverse effects, including peripheral neuropathy, headache, fatigue, vertigo, mental status changes, tremor, seizures, and GI adverse effects. • Monitor renal function test results.
pentamidine	May increase risk of pancreatitis.	• Don't use together. • If using parenteral pentamidine, don't give zalcitabine for 1 to 2 wk after stopping pentamidine.

zidovudine (AZT) • Retrovir

acyclovir	May cause severe drowsiness and lethargy.	• Acyclovir dosage may need to be reduced or stopped.
drugs that are nephrotoxic or affect bone marrow function or formation of bone marrow elements (such as amphotericin B, dapsone, doxorubicin, flucytosine, ganciclovir, interferon, pentamidine, vinblastine, vincristine)	May increase risk of toxicity of these drugs.	• Don't use with ganciclovir, if possible. • Use with other drugs cautiously. • Monitor renal function and hematologic test results closely.
probenecid	May impair elimination of zidovudine. Patient may experience malaise, myalgia, fever, and skin lesions.	• Monitor patient for these adverse effects.

zileuton • Zyflo Filmtab

drugs metabolized by the CYP3A4 isoenzyme (cyclosporine, dihydropyridine calcium channel blockers, estradiol, ethinyl, prednisone)	No formal interaction studies have been conducted.	• Give with caution. • Monitor patient for expected clinical effects and potential for increased adverse effects.
beta blockers propranolol	May increase beta-blocker effect.	• Monitor patient for increased effects (bradycardia, hypotension). • Beta blocker dose may need to be reduced.
theophylline	May decrease theophylline clearance (on average, serum theophylline level doubles).	• Monitor serum theophylline level closely; dosage adjustment may be needed, to avoid toxicity. Signs of toxicity include tachycardia, nausea, vomiting, diarrhea, restlessness, headaches, agitation, palpitations, and arrhythmias.
warfarin	May increase PT and INR.	• Monitor PT and INR; anticoagulant dose may need to be adjusted.

Interacting agents in **bold type** indicate severe, well-documented interactions.   †Canadian

INTERACTING AGENTS	POSSIBLE EFFECTS	NURSING CONSIDERATIONS
zolmitriptan • Zomig, Zomig-ZMT		
cimetidine	May double half-life of zolmitriptan.	• Monitor patient closely for increased adverse effects. • Dosage adjustments may be needed.
ergot-containing drugs	May cause additive vasospastic reactions.	• Don't give zolmitriptan within 24 hr of ergot alkaloid administration.
fluoxetine fluvoxamine paroxetine sertraline	May cause weakness, hyperreflexia, and incoordination.	• Use together cautiously. • Monitor patient for these adverse effects if used together.
MAO inhibitors	May increase plasma level of zolmitriptan.	• Monitor zolmitriptan levels; dosage adjustment may be needed. • Monitor patient for increased adverse effects. • Avoid use of drug within 2 wk of stopping MAO inhibitor therapy.
oral contraceptives	May increase mean plasma level of zolmitriptan.	• Monitor patient for increased adverse effects. Dosage adjustment may be needed.
sibutramine	May increase risk of serotonin syndrome (altered mental status; increased muscle tone, weakness, twitching; hyperthermia; delirium; coma; death).	• Don't use together.

Normal laboratory test values

Hematology
Activated partial thromboplastin time
25 to 36 seconds

Hematocrit
Men: 42% to 54%
Women: 38% to 46%

Hemoglobin, total
Men: 14 to 18 g/dl
Women: 12 to 16 g/dl

Platelet count
140,000 to 400,000/mm³

Prothrombin time
10 to 14 seconds; INR for patients on warfarin therapy, 2 to 3 (those with pediatric heart valve, 2.5 to 3.5)

Red blood cell (RBC) count
Men: 4.5 to 6.2 million/mm³ venous blood
Women: 4.2 to 5.4 million/mm³ venous blood

RBC indices
Mean corpuscular volume: 84 to 99 femtoliter

Mean corpuscular hemoglobin: 26 to 32 picograms/cell
Mean corpuscular hemoglobin concentration: 30 to 36 grams/deciliter

Reticulocyte count
0.5% to 2% of total RBC count

White blood cell (WBC) count
4,100 to 10,900/mm³

WBC differential, blood
Neutrophils: 47.6% to 76.8%
Lymphocytes: 16.2% to 43%
Monocytes: 0.6% to 9.6%
Eosinophils: 0.3% to 7%
Basophils: 0.3% to 2%

Blood chemistry
Alanine aminotransferase
Men: 10 to 35 units/L
Women: 9 to 24 units/L

Alkaline phosphatase, serum
Men ≥ age 19: 98 to 251 units/L
Women ages 24 to 65: 81 to 282 units/L
Women ≥ age 65: 119 to 309 units/L

Amylase, serum
Age ≥ 18: 35 to 115 units/L

Arterial blood gases
Pao₂: 75 to 100 mm Hg
Paco₂: 35 to 45 mm Hg
pH: 7.35 to 7.45
Sao₂: 94% to 100%
HCO₃⁻: 22 to 26 mEq/L

Aspartate aminotransferase
Men: 8 to 20 units/L
Women: 5 to 40 units/L

Bilirubin, serum
Adults: direct, < 0.5 mg/dl; indirect, 1.1 mg/dl

Blood urea nitrogen
8 to 20 mg/dl

Calcium, serum
Men ≥ age 22, women ≥ age 19: 8.9 to 10.1 mg/dl

Carbon dioxide, total, blood
22 to 34 mEq/L

Chloride, serum
100 to 108 mEq/L

(continued)

Creatine kinase (CK)
Total: Men ≥ age 18, 52 to 336 units/L;
women ≥ age 18, 38 to 176 units/L
CK-BB: None
CK-MB: 0 to 7 units/L
CK-MM: 5 to 70 units/L

Creatine, serum
Men: 0.2 to 0.6 mg/dl
Women: 0.6 to 1 mg/dl

Creatinine, serum
Men: 0.8 to 1.2 mg/dl
Women: 0.6 to 0.9 mg/dl

Glucose, fasting, plasma
70 to 100 mg/dl

Lactate dehydrogenase (LD)
Total: 48 to 115 IU/L
LD_1: 14% to 26%
LD_2: 29% to 39%
LD_3: 20% to 26%
LD_4: 8% to 16%
LD_5: 6% to 16%

Magnesium, serum
1.5 to 2.5 mEq/L
Atomic absorption: 1.7 to 2.1 mg/dl

Phosphates, serum
1.8 to 2.6 mEq/L
Atomic absorption: 2.5 to 4.5 mg/dl

Potassium, serum
3.8 to 5.5 mEq/L

Protein, total, serum
26.6 to 7.9 g/dl
Albumin fraction: 3.3 to 4.5 g/dl

Sodium, serum
135 to 145 mEq/L

Uric acid, serum
Men: 4.3 to 8 mg/dl
Women: 2.3 to 6 mg/dl

Therapeutic drug monitoring guidelines

The table below lists laboratory tests, therapeutic ranges, and guidelines for monitoring patient response to selected drugs.

DRUG	LABORATORY TEST MONITORED	THERAPEUTIC RANGES OF TEST	MONITORING GUIDELINES
aminoglycosides (amikacin, gentamicin, tobramycin)	Serum amikacin peak trough Serum gentamicin/ tobramycin peak trough Serum creatinine	20 to 30 mcg/ml 5 to 10 mcg/ml 4 to 8 mcg/ml 1 to 2 mcg/ml 0.6 to 1.3 mg/dl	Wait until administration of the third dose to check drug levels. Obtain blood for peak level 30 min after I.V. infusion or 60 min after I.M. administration. For trough levels, draw blood just before next dose. Notify prescriber of drug levels so that dosage may be adjusted accordingly. Recheck after three doses. Montior serum creatinine and BUN levels and urine output for signs of decreasing renal function.
amphotericin B	Serum creatinine BUN Serum electrolytes (especially potassium and magnesium) Liver function tests CBC with differential and platelets	0.6 to 1.3 mg/dl 7 to 18 mg/dl Potassium: 3.5 to 5 mEq/L Magnesium: 1.7 to 2.1 mEq/L Sodium: 135 to 145 mEq/L Chloride: 98 to 106 mEq/L * *****	Serum creatinine, BUN, and serum electrolyte levels should be monitored at least weekly during therapy. Also, blood counts and liver function tests should be monitored regularly during therapy. *(continued)*

Note: ***** For those areas marked with asterisks, the following values can be used:

Hemoglobin: Women: 12 to 16 g/dl
Men: 14 to 18 g/dl
Hematocrit: Women: 37% to 48%
Men: 42% to 52%

RBCs: 4 to 5.5 x 106/mm³
WBCs: 5 to 10 x 103/mm³
Differential: Neutrophils: 45% to 74%
Bands: 0% to 4%

Lymphocytes: 16% to 45%
Monocytes: 4% to 10%
Eosinophils: 0% to 7%
Basophils: 0% to 2%

* For those areas marked with one asterisk, the following values can be used:

ALT: 7 to 56 U/L
AST: 5 to 40 U/L

Alkaline phosphatase: 17 to 142 U/L
LD: 60 to 220 U/L

GGTP: < 40 U/L
Total bilirubin: 0.2 to 1 mg/dl

DRUG	LABORATORY TEST MONITORED	THERAPEUTIC RANGES OF TEST	MONITORING GUIDELINES
antibiotics	WBC with differential cultures and sensitivities	*****	Specimen cultures and sensitivities will determine the cause of the infection and the best treatment. Monitor WBC with differential weekly during therapy.
biguanides (metformin)	Serum creatinine Fasting serum glucose Glycosylated hemoglobin (HbA$_{1c}$) CBC	0.6 to 1.3 mg/dl 65 to 110 mg/dl 5.5 to 8.5% of total hemoglobin *****	Check renal function and hematologic effects before therapy starts and at least annually thereafter. If the patient has impaired renal function, don't use metformin because it may cause lactic acidosis. Monitor response to therapy with periodic evaluations of fasting glucose and HbA$_{1c}$. Home glucose monitoring by the patient can also be very useful.
clozapine	WBC with differential	*****	Obtain WBC with differential before therapy starts, weekly during therapy, and 4 wk after the drug is discontinued.
digoxin	Serum digoxin Serum electrolytes (especially potassium, magnesium, and calcium) Serum creatinine	0.5 to 2 ng/ml Potassium: 3.5 to 5 mEq/L Magnesium: 1.7 to 2.1 mEq/L Sodium: 135 to 145 mEq/L Chloride: 98 to 106 mEq/L Calcium: 8.6 to 10 mg/dl 0.6 to 1.3 mg/dl	Serum digoxin level should be checked at least 12 hr, but preferably 24 hr, after the last dose is given. For monitoring maintenance therapy, levels should be checked at least 2 wk after therapy starts or changes. Adjustments in therapy should be made based on entire clinical picture, not solely on drug levels. Electrolytes and renal function should also be checked periodically during therapy.
diuretics	Serum electrolytes	Potassium: 3.5 to 5 mEq/L Magnesium: 1.7 to 2.1 mEq/L Sodium: 135 to 145 mEq/L Chloride: 98 to 106 mEq/L Calcium: 8.6 to 10 mg/dl	To monitor fluid and electrolyte balance, baseline and periodic determinations of serum electrolytes, serum calcium, BUN, uric acid, and serum glucose levels should be performed.

	Serum creatinine	0.6 to 1.3 mg/dl	
	BUN	7 to 18 mg/dl	
	Uric acid	2 to 7 mg/dl	
	Fasting serum glucose	65 to 110 mg/dl	
erythropoietin	Hematocrit	Women: 36% to 48% Men: 42% to 52%	After therapy starts or changes, monitor hematocrit twice weekly for 2 to 6 wk until stabilized in the target range and a maintenance dosage is determined. The hematocrit should be monitored at regular intervals thereafter.
ethosuximide	Serum ethosuximide	40 to 100 mcg/ml	Check level 10 to 13 days after therapy starts or changes.
gemfibrozil	Serum lipids	Total cholesterol: < 200 mg/dl LDL: < 130 mg/dl HDL: women: 40 to 85 mg/dl men: 37 to 70 mg/dl Triglycerides: 40 to 160 mg/dl	Therapy is usually withdrawn after 3 mo if response isn't adequate. Patient must be fasting to measure triglycerides.
heparin	Activated partial thromboplastin time (aPTT)	1.5 to 2 times control	When drug is given by continuous I.V. infusion, aPTT should be checked every 4 hr in the early stages of therapy. When given by deep S.C. injection, aPTT should be checked 4 to 6 hr after injection. *(continued)*

Note: ***** For those areas marked with asterisks, the following values can be used:

Hemoglobin: Women: 12 to 16 g/dl
  Men: 14 to 18 g/dl
Hematocrit: Women: 37% to 48%
  Men: 42% to 52%

RBCs: 4 to 5.5 x 10⁶/mm³
WBCs: 5 to 10 x 10³/mm³
Differential: Neutrophils: 45% to 74%
  Bands: 0% to 4%

Lymphocytes: 16% to 45%
Monocytes: 4% to 10%
Eosinophils: 0% to 7%
Basophils: 0% to 2%

* For those areas marked with one asterisk, the following values can be used:

ALT: 7 to 56 U/L
AST: 5 to 40 U/L

Alkaline phosphatase: 17 to 142 U/L
LD: 60 to 220 U/L

GGTP: < 40 U/L
Total bilirubin: 0.2 to 1 mg/dl

DRUG	LABORATORY TEST MONITORED	THERAPEUTIC RANGES OF TEST	MONITORING GUIDELINES
HMG-CoA reductase inhibitors (fluvastatin, lovastatin, pravastatin, simvastatin)	Serum lipids Liver function tests	Total cholesterol: < 200 mg/dl LDL: < 130 mg/dl HDL: women: 40 to 85 mg/dl men: 37 to 70 mg/dl Triglycerides: 40 to 160 mg/dl *	Liver function tests should be determined at baseline, 6 to 12 wk after therapy starts or changes, and periodically thereafter. If adequate response isn't achieved within 6 wk, a change in therapy should be considered.
insulin	Fasting serum glucose HbA$_{1c}$	65 to 110 mg/dl 5.5% to 8.5% of total hemoglobin	Monitor response to therapy with evaluations of serum glucose and HbA$_{1c}$. Glycosylated hemoglobin is a good measure of long-term control. Home glucose monitoring by the patient is also useful for measuring compliance and response.
lithium	Serum lithium Serum creatinine CBC Serum electrolytes (especially potassium and sodium) Fasting serum glucose Thyroid function tests	0.6 to 1.2 mEq/L 0.6 to 1.3 mg/dl * * * * * Potassium: 3.5 to 5 mEq/L Magnesium: 1.7 to 2.1 mEq/L Sodium: 135 to 145 mEq/L Chloride: 98 to 106 mEq/L 65 to 110 mg/dl TSH: 0.2 to 5.4 microU/mL T$_3$: 80 to 200 ng/ml T$_4$: 5.4 to 11.5 mcg/dl	Checking serum lithium level is crucial to the safe use of the drug. Obtain serum lithium level immediately before next dose. Levels should be monitored twice weekly until stable. Once at steady state, levels may be obtained weekly; when the patient is on the appropriate maintenance dosage, levels may be monitored every 2 to 3 mo. Monitor serum creatinine, serum electrolyte, and fasting serum glucose levels; CBC; and thyroid function tests as needed, before therapy starts and periodically during therapy.
methotrexate	Serum methotrexate	Normal elimination: < 10 micromol 24 hours post dose < 1 micromol 48 hours post dose	Methotrexate level should be monitored according to dosing protocol. CBC with differential and platelet count, and liver and renal function tests should be monitored more frequently when therapy starts or changes and when methotrexate level may be ele-

		< 0.2 micromol 72 hours post dose *****	vated (such as in dehydration).
	CBC with differential		
	Platelet count	140 to 400 x 10³/mm³	
	Liver function tests	*	
	Serum creatinine	0.6 to 1.3 mg/dl	
phenytoin	Serum phenytoin	10 to 20 mcg/ml	Serum phenytoin level should be monitored immediately before next dose, 2 to 4 wk after therapy starts or dosage is adjusted. A CBC should be obtained at baseline and monthly early in therapy. Notify prescriber if toxic effects appear at therapeutic levels. The measured level should be adjusted for hypoalbuminemia or renal impairment, which can increase free drug levels.
	CBC	*****	
potassium chloride	Serum potassium	3.5 to 5 mEq/L	Check level weekly after oral replacement therapy starts until stable, and every 3 to 6 mo thereafter.
procainamide	Serum procainamide	4 to 8 mcg/ml (procainamide)	Procainamide level should be measured 6 to 12 hr after a continuous infusion starts, or immediately before the next oral dose. Combined (procainamide and NAPA) levels can be used as an index of toxicity when renal impairment exists. CBC should be obtained periodically during longer-term therapy.
	Serum N-acetylpro-cainamide	5 to 30 mcg/ml (combined procainamide and NAPA)	
	CBC	*****	*(continued)*

Note: ***** For those areas marked with asterisks, the following values can be used:

Hemoglobin: Women: 12 to 16 g/dl
Men: 14 to 18 g/dl
Hematocrit: Women: 37% to 48%
Men: 42% to 52%

RBCs: 4 to 5.5 x 10⁶/mm³
WBCs: 5 to 10 x 10³/mm³
Differential: Neutrophils: 45% to 74%
Bands: 0% to 4%

Lymphocytes: 16% to 45%
Monocytes: 4% to 10%
Eosinophils: 0% to 7%
Basophils: 0% to 2%

* For those areas marked with one asterisk, the following values can be used:

ALT: 7 to 56 U/L
AST: 5 to 40 U/L

Alkaline phosphatase: 17 to 142 U/L
LD: 60 to 220 U/L

GGTP: < 40 U/L
Total bilirubin: 0.2 to 1 mg/dl

DRUG	LABORATORY TEST MONITORED	THERAPEUTIC RANGES OF TEST	MONITORING GUIDELINES
quinidine	Serum quinidine CBC Liver function tests Serum creatinine Serum electrolytes (especially potassium)	2 to 6 mcg/ml ***** * 0.6 to 1.3 mg/dl Potassium: 3.5 to 5 mEq/L Magnesium: 1.7 to 2.1 mEq/L Sodium: 135 to 145 mEq/L Chloride: 98 to 106 mEq/L	Levels should be obtained immediately before next oral dose, 30 to 35 hr after therapy starts or dosage is changed. Blood counts, liver and kidney function tests, and serum electrolyte levels should be obtained peroidically.
sulfonylureas	Fasting serum glucose HbA_{1c}	65 to 110 mg/dl 5.8% to 8.5% of total hemoglobin	Response to therapy should be monitored with periodic evaluations of fasting glucose and HbA_{1c}. Home glucose monitoring by the patient is a good measure of compliance and response.
theophylline	Serum theophylline	10 to 20 mcg/ml	Serum theophylline level should be obtained immediately before next dose of sustained-release oral product, at least 2 days after therapy starts or changes.
thyroid hormone	Thyroid function tests	TSH: 0.2 to 5.4 microU/ml T_3: 80 to 200 ng/dl T_4: 5.4 to 11.5 mcg/dl	Thyroid function tests should be monitored every 2 to 3 wk until appropriate maintenance dosage is determined.
vancomycin	Serum vancomycin Serum creatinine	20 to 40 mcg/ml (peak) 5 to 10 mcg/ml (trough) 0.6 to 1.3 mg/dl	Serum vancomycin level may be checked when the third dose is given (at the earliest). Peak levels should be drawn ½ hr after the completion of an I.V. infusion. Trough levels should be drawn immediately before the next dose is given. Renal function can be used to adjust dosing and intervals.
warfarin	INR	For acute MI; atrial fibrillation; treatment of pulmonary embolism; prevention of	Daily INR should be obtained beginning 3 days after therapy starts and continuing until therapeutic goal is achieved, with periodic monitoring thereafter.

systemic embolism, tissue heart valves, valvular heart disease; or prophylaxis or treatment of venous thrombosis: 2 to 3

For mechanical prosthetic valves or recurrent systemic embolism: 3 to 4.5

Levels should also be checked 7 days after any change in warfarin dose or potentially interacting therapy.

Note: ***** For those areas marked with asterisks, the following values can be used:

Hemoglobin: Women: 12 to 16 g/dl
  Men: 14 to 18 g/dl
Hematocrit: Women: 37% to 48%
  Men: 42% to 52%

RBCs: 4 to 5.5 x 106/mm³
WBCs: 5 to 10 x 103/mm³
Differential: Neutrophils: 45% to 74%
  Bands: 0% to 4%

Lymphocytes: 16% to 45%
Monocytes: 4% to 10%
Eosinophils: 0% to 7%
Basophils: 0% to 2%

* For those areas marked with one asterisk, the following values can be used:

ALT: 7 to 56 U/L
AST: 5 to 40 U/L

Alkaline phosphatase: 17 to 142 U/L
LD: 60 to 220 U/L

GGTP: < 40 U/L
Total bilirubin: 0.2 to 1 mg/dl

Index

G

O

W